Social Factors in the Personality Disorders

Second Edition

Social Factors in the Personality Disorders

Finding a Niche

Second Edition

Joel Paris
McGill University

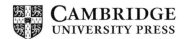

CAMBRIDGE
UNIVERSITY PRESS

University Printing House, Cambridge CB2 8BS, United Kingdom

One Liberty Plaza, 20th Floor, New York, NY 10006, USA

477 Williamstown Road, Port Melbourne, VIC 3207, Australia

314–321, 3rd Floor, Plot 3, Splendor Forum, Jasola District Centre,
New Delhi – 110025, India

79 Anson Road, #06–04/06, Singapore 079906

Cambridge University Press is part of the University of Cambridge.

It furthers the University's mission by disseminating knowledge in the pursuit of
education, learning, and research at the highest international levels of excellence.

www.cambridge.org
Information on this title: www.cambridge.org/9781108811637
DOI: 10.1017/9781108867542

First published 2020

Printed in the United Kingdom by TJ International Ltd, Padstow Cornwall

A catalogue record for this publication is available from the British Library.

Library of Congress Cataloging-in-Publication Data
Names: Paris, Joel, 1940- author.
Title: Social factors in the personality disorders : finding a niche / Joel Paris.
Description: Second edition. | New York : Cambridge University Press, 2020. |
   Includes bibliographical references and index.
Identifiers: LCCN 2020009236 (print) | LCCN 2020009237 (ebook) |
   ISBN 9781108811637 (paperback) | ISBN 9781108867542 (epub)
Subjects: LCSH: Personality disorders–Social aspects. | Personality disorders–Etiology. |
   Personality disorders–Treatment.
Classification: LCC RC554 .P37 2020 (print) | LCC RC554 (ebook) |
   DDC 616.85/81–dc23
LC record available at https://lccn.loc.gov/2020009236
LC ebook record available at https://lccn.loc.gov/2020009237

ISBN 978-1-108-81163-7 Paperback

....

Every effort has been made in preparing this book to provide accurate and up-to-date
information that is in accord with accepted standards and practice at the time of

Contents

Foreword

In 2005 I attended a meeting of the American Psychiatric Association (APA) in which the term "biopsychosocial model" of mental illness came up frequently in the preamble to the presentations. However, the president of the APA at that time, Dr. Steven Sharfstein, was far from pleased. He complained that most of the presentations at the meeting were about the "bio-bio-bio model" – they were neglecting the psychological and social aspects in favor of the medical ones. His words had an impact; much has changed since. At least this overbiological slant of 2005 could never be said of this book on the social aspects of personality disorders. Moreover, Dr. Paris has cleverly avoided the trap of being one-sided and overegging the social aspects. Here he is not pushing the social-social model or even the trauma-trauma model of personality dysfunction. He covers everything you need to know: the genetics, the biological aspects, the environmental and social factors, the etiological precursors of personality disorder and its progress over time.

The first edition of this book in 1996 had "biopsychosocial" in its subtitle but much has happened in the field in the last quarter century to show that even this term, rather a clumsy one, is now outdated. Dr. Paris's book shows the interaction of not just the biopsychosocial aspects of personality but also gene–environment interplay, evolutionary aspects, and both sociological and political elements. I would prefer to say this book is a protagonist of the "omnirerum (or omnireric) model", a model of mental disorders that is comprehensive and all-embracing. After reading you can appreciate that personality function is extraordinarily fluid. At times it dominates functioning and can be very damaging, yet at others it integrates and holds people together, its genetic and environmental elements working in harmony. The dichotomous notion of personality disorder versus nondisorder is shown by Dr. Paris to be ludicrous; the combination of personality attributes makes the whole world kin. It is only when the combination locks in programs of maladjusted error that disorder is shown.

This book is both a reference text and an inspiration for future developments. It is also optimistic. It shows that personality disorder is not a permanent stain on the psyche. It is just as changeable as other mental illness, and this needs more emphasis, over and over again to those of our prejudiced colleagues who regularly avoid the term. I consider the most important sentence in the book is one from the last chapter:

" The most important clinical implication of the model lies in helping patients finding a niche in the social world. No matter what personality traits you have, they can be modified to promote functioning in society, work, and relationships."

Nevertheless, I have to declare an interest here. In this sentence Dr. Paris is describing the essential message of nidotherapy in the management of all personality disorders, and if you wish to know more you might want to look into the subject further (Tyrer & Tyrer, 2018). However, be sure to read this book from cover to cover first.

Peter Tyrer
Emeritus Professor of Community Psychiatry, Imperial College, London
January 2020

Preface to the Second Edition

A quarter-century has elapsed since the first edition of this book was published. Since then an enormous body of research has appeared concerning biological and psychological risk factors for personality disorders (PDs), as well as for biological and psychological methods of treatment. However, less attention has been paid to the social context of PDs, i.e., how personality traits and disorders interact with social demands and opportunities. Yet social forces carry important risks for the development of PDs.

This second edition will be briefer and more focused than the previous one. I have not included a good deal of material that was in the first edition, addressing the psychological roots of PDs, and describing their treatment in some detail. These issues have been discussed in many other books, including several that I have written. I wanted this new edition to have a more consistent focus on social risk factors that, in interaction with biological and psychological risks, can determine whether or not people who have these risks go on to develop diagnosable disorders. I also wanted to show that social forces have clinical relevance, in that they determine whether people with different traits can find a niche in life.

Personality disorders are rooted in personality traits. We all have a personality. But it need not become disordered if we can find a social *niche* that fits our particular characteristics. If we do not find that niche, then psychopathology is more likely to ensue. That is one of the main themes of this new edition.

The argument of this book will be backed up by research. Personality traits are heritable variants that lie within a normal range: adaptive under some circumstances but maladaptive under others. About half of the variance in personality and PDs is under genetic influence. Levels of psychosocial risk are complex: some derive from dysfunctional families, but most of the variance is not related to growing up in a specific family. The larger social environment plays a crucial role of its own.

Consider some examples. People with emotionally unstable and impulsive traits may be at risk for PDs, such as borderline personality disorder (BPD), when environmental circumstances are adverse. But when circumstances are favorable, they can use the same traits to become productive and energetic members of society. People who are unusually self-centered can turn their traits into ambition and productivity, but can also develop into unlovable narcissists. People who are socially anxious may find life niches that do not demand high levels of interaction, and that favor introversion. This allows them to avoid the instability seen in other personality types, but can also make them suffer from loneliness and isolation.

This book will show that social factors are important in PDs, will support a biopsychosocial model of these disorders, and will review empirical evidence substantiating it. It will also include new separate chapters on borderline, narcissistic, and antisocial PDs. It will further develop a model that takes into account social change and the social stressors that interfere with finding a niche in the world. The new edition will also develop a more general theory of how social networks and social capital influence personality functioning. Finally, this revision will show how this view of personality and PDs is relevant to clinical practice.

Introduction

The Origins of This Book

The treatment of patients with personality disorders (PDs) can be arduous, and is not always successful. It should therefore be no surprise that therapists working with this population look for advice. Yet there are limits to the value of expert opinion.

As a student, I was taught that PDs derive largely from negative childhood experiences. Readers of this book may be surprised how weak the evidence is for this conclusion. At best, the idea that the etiology of PDs is mainly the result of psychological adversity is a half-truth. At worst, it is a misleading oversimplification of a complex issue. Childhood adversity is a risk factor, but does not necessarily, by itself, lead to a disordered personality. Also, not every patient with a PD will have had a troubled childhood.

These discrepancies can be partly accounted for by evidence that PDs are moderately heritable. In this respect, PDs can be exaggerations of genetic predispositions. However, that is also by no means the whole story. Today many clinicians believe that the future of research and practice lies with genes, biomarkers, and errant neural connections. Nevertheless, while neuroscience may eventually illuminate the problems of PDs, its relevance to practice remains a long way off.

What is missing from this picture? Both early adversity and heritable predispositions are *risk factors* for psychopathology, but are not causes. Neither are consistent predictors for the emergence of any mental disorder. We need a gene–environment model of PD, a theory that describes how temperament and adverse environments interact. We also need to understand that people who develop PDs are not isolated individuals. Like the rest of us, they are subject to powerful social forces. In addition, the modern world is particularly challenging for people with trait vulnerabilities.

Finally, while efficacious psychotherapy is now available for some categories of PD (especially borderline personality disorder, or BPD), they are not useful for all patients. Also, there are no consistently effective medications for PDs; even if they were possible, they remain to be invented.

Thus, those who believe that PDs are rooted in abnormalities of the connectome, or in adverse childhood environments, are taking ideological positions. There is little evidence that PDs can be treated successfully with biological interventions alone, or by psychotherapies that focus on digging up the past.

Why I Have Written This Book

This troubling gap between research and practice parallels the trajectory of my own career. Fifty years ago, I entered training to be a clinical psychiatrist, with a particular interest in psychotherapy. I spent much of the first 10 years after residency treating PD patients. Working in a clinic at a teaching hospital, I taught students to evaluate and manage this population.

Like most clinicians, my own results as a therapist varied from gratifying success to complete failure, with most cases falling somewhere between. At first, I assumed that I lacked sufficient experience. Eventually I realized that my teachers had not told me the truth. In spite of their longer experience, their results were no better than mine.

I then came to realize the need for a better theory to explain the difficulties with which my patients and I must grapple. Until we know more, we cannot expect to treat PDs with greater success. I also concluded that we would never succeed in understanding the etiology of PDs by collecting more clinical material, and by theorizing from the armchair. The subject demanded systematic empirical investigation.

These reflections led me to develop a second career as a researcher. I was fortunate enough to find colleagues who were interested in the same questions, and with whom I worked to collect data on the etiology of the personality disorders, and on their outcome. Research experiences changed my attitudes as a clinician. I became converted to the principles of "evidence-based medicine". I came to believe that, as much as possible, treatment should be based on empirical data and the evidence of clinical trials.

But therapists can hardly afford to wait 50 years until adequate empirical knowledge is collected to support practice. We are faced every day with troubled patients who have a legitimate need for help. We must do our best for them until more evidence is forthcoming. Clinicians need to be humble, given the serious methodological and logistic problems that inevitably arise in the study of highly complex disorders.

This book will present a general model of PD etiology that takes social risk factors into account. I will discuss these mechanisms in terms of interactions between biological, psychological, and social risks, and show how they can be integrated in a multidimensional model. I will then suggest that the most important clinical implication of the model lies in helping patients finding a niche in the social world. No matter what personality traits you have, they can be modified to promote functioning in society, work, and relationships.

Part I

General Principles

Personality Disorders
The History of an Idea

Personality disorders (PDs) were not always considered to be mental illnesses. Even today, there is resistance to this point of view. So how did people with these problems come to be seen as meriting a psychiatric diagnosis? The problem has always concerned how to draw a line between normality and pathology.

All medical illnesses lie on a continuum with normality. The determination of what is a "case" is in many respects a social construct (Eisenberg, 1986, 1995). Some patients might be considered unwise or unlucky in love, while others are seen as "more bad than mad". What justifies seeing people with diagnosable PDs as having mental disorders is that they have serious exaggerations of normal personality traits. At some point, these amplifications produce significant levels of dysfunction that can be considered pathological.

The acceptance of PDs as valid diagnoses reflected a change in psychiatric ideology. During most of history, mental illness was synonymous with "madness", i.e., psychosis or severe depression. However, there has been a consistent expansion of the construct of mental disorders. To understand the historical context of this change, let us first have a look at the history of how personality and PDs have been seen in the past.

Personality and Personality Disorder in Historical Context
The classification of personality (as opposed to PD) has a long history that can be traced back to the Greeks (Butcher, 2010). A theory describing four temperaments (choleric, sanguine, phlegmatic, and melancholic) was associated with the Roman physician Galen (Kagan, 1994) and dominated thinking about personality for many centuries. Even today, if one considers Galen's temperamental types as descriptors (ignoring anachronistic physiological speculations), his four temperaments can be considered as precursors of trait theories.

Throughout most of history differences in these temperamental types were considered to be variants of normal personality, lying outside the purview of psychiatry. In the 19th century, physicians recognized only one form of pathological personality as a diagnosis. They termed this entity "moral insanity", defined by an inability to control criminal actions, i.e., today's antisocial personality or psychopathy (Berrios, 1993).

The gradual acceptance of PDs as valid diagnoses over the next hundred years also reflected a broadening scope of practice. In the early part of the 19th century, psychiatry was based in mental hospitals, and concerned itself almost exclusively with psychoses. The construct of "moral insanity" appeared at a time when the field was expanding. Medical specialists might now be consulted in criminal cases, and patients in psychiatric hospitals were no longer exclusively psychotic. Yet in the course of the 19th century, as the major forms of mental disorder were reclassified, influential theoreticians (e.g., Kraepelin, 1919) hypothesized that pathological forms of personality are occult forms of psychosis.

By the beginning of the 20th century, psychiatrists no longer restricted themselves to treatment of severe mental disorders, but moved clinical practice from hospitals into outpatient clinics and private offices. Many clinicians became interested in understanding problems in interpersonal relationships and in treating these life problems with psychotherapy. Their practice profile largely consisted of patients who would, today, be classified as suffering from PDs.

In the 20th century, psychoanalysis became a driving force behind the acceptance of PDs. Ironically, analysts were not at first interested in personality, but focused on the treatment of symptomatic neuroses. Since they tended to assume that the personality behind symptoms remained intact, their therapies were brief and not geared to characterological change. Yet, over time, psychoanalytically oriented clinicians came to view all psychiatric symptoms as rooted in personality. However, experience with analytic methods showed that symptoms were not easily removed and personality was not easily changed, even with increasingly lengthy treatment.

In the postwar heyday of psychoanalysis in North America, characterological change became a main goal of analytic therapy (Hale, 1995). Paradoxically, the success of biological psychiatrists in treating symptomatic neuroses with drugs reinforced this trend, leaving personality disorders as a residual domain for psychotherapy.

Wilhelm Reich (1933/1990) was the first psychoanalyst to develop an explicit method for treating character pathology. He described the function of maladaptive personality as "character armor", by which he meant that personality traits protect the patient against neurotic symptoms. This theory was a forerunner of the modern construct of defense mechanisms. Reich thought that if the therapist could remove character armor, the patient would experience symptoms that could then be more readily treated. If personality traits were "egosyntonic", i.e., not seen by patients as a problem, they might require some form of "character analysis".

Since most European psychoanalysts were forced to emigrate to North America for political reasons, the 1930s and 1940s were a period when the sociopolitical climate had a strong influence on psychological theories. Some analysts were interested in understanding personality pathology in a social context. Karen Horney (1940), combining clinical observations with social criticism, suggested that excessive individualism in Western culture was a cause of "neurotic personality". Erich Fromm (1955), a committed socialist, thought that neurotic personality structures reflected excessively acquisitive economic behavior associated with capitalism.

The transplantation of analysis across the Atlantic converted it from a conservative European idea into an environmental American theory (Torrey, 1992). Europeans, with their strong historical traditions, may be more likely to believe that personality is fixed. Americans are descended from immigrants who rejected Europe to start anew, and therefore are more likely to believe in the importance of the environment.

During the period before World War II, European psychiatry took a very different direction from ideas prevalent in North America. Psychoanalytic theories of the etiology of mental illness were not generally accepted. Mental disorders were seen as largely determined by constitutional factors. The leading European psychiatrists were not interested in looking for putative psychological causes, but in using systematic phenomenological observations to classify mental disorders.

Kurt Schneider (1950) developed a classification system for the personality disorders that was influential in Europe. He defined ten forms of "psycho-pathic personality", each with specific behavioral patterns. His categories resembled those later developed for the *Diagnostic and Statistical Manual of Mental Disorders* (DSM) and earlier *International Classification of Diseases* (ICD) classifications.

During the postwar period, theoretical differences created a divergence in psychiatric classification between North America and Europe. DSM-I (American Psychiatric Association, 1952) was influenced by the ideas of the Swiss-born psychiatrist Adolf Meyer (1957). Meyer saw psychopathology not as a set of disease categories, but of reaction patterns. Although he accepted in principle that biological factors influence predispositions to mental illness, in practice Meyer was environmentally oriented, with a theory that strongly emphasized psychosocial factors. In this respect, Meyerian "psychobiology" was typically American.

DSM-II (American Psychiatric Association, 1968) made an effort to ensure American classification accorded with international standards, creating categories of personality disorders more similar to those described in ICD. However, its approach to the classification of PDs was no better than in the previous edition.

European phenomenological traditions emphasize the clinical symptoms of mental illness, postponing etiological speculation until hard data becomes available. This approach eventually gained popularity across the Atlantic, due to a reaction against the excesses of psychoanalytic speculation, as well as the inefficiency of psychodynamic therapies. At this point, the classification of PDs in the earlier editions of DSM were fairly primitive, and no research was conducted to find out the causes of PDs, or what might help patients with these conditions. Moreover, while psychoanalysis had proclaimed itself to be a comprehensive theory of mental illness, as well as an effective treatment for a wide range of mentally disordered patients, it became increasingly obvious that there was no scientific basis for either of these claims.

Social and historical factors have influenced the dominance of the psychodynamic approach in American psychiatry. In the postwar political climate, North Americans were isolated from European thought. Americans can be idealistic, tending to be suspicious of constitutional theories of human nature and preferring to believe that new beginnings in life are always possible. For this reason, theoretical developments in biology, such as ethology and sociobiology, emphasizing the strong influence of genes on human behavior, caused little controversy in Europe, but became the target of opposition in America (Barkow et al., 1992).

Seventy years ago, it was possible to train in psychiatry in North America and to be unfamiliar with the work of Emil Kraepelin. However, the field was about to fall under the influence of "neo-Kraepelinian" theory (Klerman, 1986). The reason was that psychiatrists became committed to developing an empirical base for their specialty. The neo-Kraepelinian group was centered in the Midwest, where psychoanalytic ideas had never been as popular as in coastal regions. This movement was the conceptual basis of DSM-III (American Psychiatric Association, 1980).

DSM-III was a diagnostic system that used observable criteria to operationalize all constructs, including personality disorders. While it may be radically revised in the future, its categorical classification of PDs was retained in DSM-5 (albeit offering an alternative – see Chapter 2).

With empiricism dominating American psychiatry, psychoanalysis was displaced and left in a peripheral role. Since the concept of PD was clearly rooted in a model that cannot be considered a scientific theory, it met with resistance. Yet biological psychiatry, which now became the dominant paradigm, also had limitations. Neuroscience takes a reductionistic approach, in which neuronal connections are seen as more "real" than broader concepts of mind or personality. While there has always been a literature on social factors in mental disorders, this aspect tends to be sidelined.

Several of the founders of research on personality disorders were psychotherapists who chose to enter the empirical mainstream and study PDs with empirical methods. One of the most prominent examples was John

Gunderson (Gunderson & Singer, 1975), a psychoanalyst with a research training, who showed how the construct of borderline personality disorder (BPD) could be measured in the same way as other mental disorders. Later, analysts such as Anthony Bateman and Peter Fonagy (2004) also made major research contributions to the understanding of PDs.

Cognitive behaviorally oriented psychotherapists have also contributed to the development of research on PDs. Aaron Beck, the founder of cognitive behavioral therapy (CBT), is the co-author of several editions of a textbook about treating PDs (Beck & Freeman, 2015). However, the most important figure coming out of this tradition is Marsha Linehan (1993), a psychologist who taught a generation of clinicians the crucial role of emotion regulation in etiology and treatment. Her method for BPD, dialectical behavior therapy (DBT), became a gold standard for many therapists.

Another stream of ideas, derived from trait psychology, has also influenced the way we think about PDs. Academic psychologists have long been involved in the measurement of personality traits, using factor analysis of data from self-report questionnaires. This psychometric tradition can be applied to the domains of personality. The result is a "dimensional" approach to personality disorders. The most important current system is the Five Factor Model (Costa & Widiger, 2013), which will be examined in more detail in Chapter 2.

Why Social Risk Factors Are Often Ignored

The recognition of the importance of social factors in mental illness goes back to Emil Durkheim (1897/1997), the pioneer sociologist whose ideas continue to influence mental health professionals. His work on the relationship of society to suicide remains seminal.

Yet, the relationship between sociology and psychiatry has often been uneasy and distant (Morgan & Kleinman, 2010). This is due partly to attacks by hostile sociologists such as Scheff (1989) who argued that mental illness does not exist, and represents little but social deviance. This schism has been magnified by the biological paradigm that currently dominates psychiatry, in which social factors are not seriously considered (Paris, 2008).

A sociologist who is sympathetic to psychiatry (Horwitz, 2002) has observed that the current classification of mental disorders assumes the reality of its categories, fails to take social context into account, and expands the range of psychopathology into normal human experience. This is a fair critique, but social psychiatry also needs to prove its case – by conducting its own clinical trials to show that interventions derived from sociological theory are effective in practice.

Unfortunately, social factors in mental disorders continue to go unrecognized. Many patients who see psychiatrists only have medications prescribed, adjusted, or changed. In addition, they do not often receive evidence-based psychotherapy (Olfson et al., 2002). A point of view that fails to consider the social context of symptoms has taken hold. Even in severe mental illnesses such as schizophrenia, bipolar-I disorder, or melancholic depression, a purely biological approach fails to address psychosocial issues that can interfere with recovery (Topor et al., 2011).

In short, biological psychiatry is too narrow a paradigm to account for all mental disorders. A specialty that defines itself as the clinical application of neuroscience, as suggested by Insel and Quirion (2005) ends up with a "mindless" point of view, reducing complex psychosocial phenomena to a neuronal level. The model is even less appropriate for common mental disorders such as mild to moderate depression (Kirsch et al., 2008), or anxiety disorders (Otto et al., 2006), in which medication often has inconsistent effects.

A purely neuroscience-based model is particularly problematic for understanding or treating patients with personality disorders, who do not respond in any consistent way to antidepressants (Newton-Jones et al., 2006) or to any other currently available medication (Stoffers et al., 2010).

Personality Disorders in Social Context

The dominance of biological psychiatry, associated with the decline of a psychosocial perspective, has marginalized the understanding of PDs. Modern psychiatry, with its focus on symptoms, is not interested in personality and therefore tends to miss these diagnoses entirely or consider them as secondary or "comorbid".

Yet PD can be the primary diagnosis in patients who have had a troubled life over many years, and the construct describes their dysfunction more comprehensively (American Psychiatric Association, 2013). Taking personality into account requires clinicians to go beyond symptoms, obtain a life history, and examine trajectories of psychosocial functioning over time. That kind of assessment goes against the current trend to train clinicians to concentrate on symptoms and on interventions that reduce symptoms. Often, patients are only referred to specialists after the failure of pharmacological therapy. Yet there is good evidence that psychotherapy specifically designed for PDs can be effective (Paris, 2010a).

A social perspective is also necessary for understanding how disorders develop and how patients recover from them. While research on PDs has advanced in recent decades, little attention has been paid to their social context. Only a few theorists (Millon, 1993; Paris, 1996) have focused on the impact of social stressors, and only a few studies (Walsh et al., 2012) have formally measured them.

Variations in personality traits reflect alternative behavioral strategies that can be adaptive or maladaptive, depending on environmental conditions (Beck & Freeman, 2015). The traits underlying PDs can be functional in some contexts but not others. Thus antisocial traits such as fearlessness could be adaptive in soldiers, while avoidant traits need not be pathological in cultures where social roles and marital partners are provided by society.

One of the most important social stressors in modern societies derives from cultural variations concerning values of individualism or collectivism, which can be associated with either normative or pathological outcomes in different societies (Caldwell-Harris & Aycicegi, 2006). Modern societies, because of their high demand for individuality, create difficulties for people with a strong need for social support (Paris, 2013). There is some evidence that antisocial personality disorder (ASPD), BPD (Millon, 1993), as well as narcissistic personality disorder (NPD) (Twenge & Campbell, 2009) are increasing in prevalence. All these PDs, marked by impulsivity, emerge in an individualistic culture that rewards risk-taking but fails to provide emotional support. Similarly, disorders associated with high introversion, such as avoidant PD, may arise in societies that expect high levels of autonomy (which not everyone can attain).

In summary, PD, an amalgam of temperament, life experience, and social context, is quintessentially *biopsychosocial*. This book will aim to go beyond the lip service so often given to that concept and examine how social factors interact with biological and psychological risks in etiology and treatment.

Personality Traits and Personality Disorders

The Nature and Origin of Personality Traits

Every individual has a set of unique behavioral characteristics, popularly called "personality". These *traits* are consistent patterns of behavior, emotion, and cognition. Traits vary greatly between individuals, can be identified early in life, and are fairly stable over time. The broadest characteristics of personality do not change in any dramatic way between the ages of 18 and 60 (Costa & Widiger, 2013).

Both genetic and environmental factors play a role in shaping personality. Thus Rutter (1987) suggested that two factors influence trait profiles: temperament and social learning. Temperament describes behavioral dispositions present at birth. Observations of newborn infants show that they differ from each other in how active they are, in how sociable they are, in how easily they get upset, and in how readily they can calm down (Kagan, 1994; Rothbart, 2011).

Moreover, temperamental effects need not be limited to characteristics present at birth, since a number of genetic effects on personality only "switch on" at later periods of development (Rutter, 2006). Most children with a moderately difficult temperament never develop mental disorders. Infantile temperament is not notably continuous with later personality, although temperamental characteristics measured later in development are more predictive of adult personality traits and functioning.

Extreme temperaments are stronger predictors of psychopathology. For example, longitudinal studies of children with high levels of shyness (Kagan, 1994) find relationships with anxious symptoms in adolescence. Although temperament "bends the twig" by setting limits on the predominant characteristics of any individual, environment plays an equally important role. Bandura (1977) hypothesized a process of learning in which behavioral patterns in children are shaped in two ways: by positive and negative reinforcement and by the modeling of behaviors that children observe in adults.

Most trait differences are entirely compatible with normality. They are generally more adaptive in some circumstances than in others. It is only when traits significantly interfere with functioning, and when behaviors are used rigidly and maladaptively, that one can speak of a personality disorder (PD).

Measuring Personality Dimensions

The traits that define individual differences in personality can be measured quantitatively. Personality as a whole can be thought of as consisting of a set of traits, the scoring of which can be pictured as a dimension in space. It is for this reason that traits are called the *dimensions* of personality.

Many personality characteristics are "egosyntonic". This means that, in contrast to symptoms that are alien to the self, or "egodystonic", egosyntonic traits are considered by those who have them as normal. For this reason, studying personality entirely through self-report presents a problem. Certain traits might not even be reported at all. There are advantages in adding observations from interviews, or data from informants. However, since interviews are cumbersome and can have problems in reliability, most of the research on personality dimensions has been carried out using self-report instruments, in which questions are cunningly designed to allow people to describe themselves in a neutral and therefore relatively accurate fashion.

The questionnaires that measure personality traits are composed of items that describe a wide range of behaviors and attitudes. The dimensions of personality are identified from these scores, using a statistical procedure called factor analysis. This method gathers together intercorrelated items on the questionnaire into "factors", which can then be labeled by describing common characteristics.

Factor analysis can either be used to describe a smaller number of broadly defined factors, or a larger number of narrowly defined factors. Therefore, dimensional models fall into two general types. A few broad dimensions or many narrow dimensions can be used to describe personality. Each method has its advantages and disadvantages. Broad dimensions are closer to temperament, but narrow dimensions, such as the "facets" of the Five Factor Model (FFM) domains (Costa & Widiger, 2013), or in other systems (e.g., Livesley et al., 1993) offer a more detailed view of personality.

Dimensional models take the position that PDs are exaggerations of normal traits. In both community and clinical populations, traits and disorders often appear to be continuous (Costa & Widiger, 2013). Personality disorders become diagnosable at a cutoff point, beyond which traits are maladaptively intense. An analogous situation would be hypertension, which is defined by a cutoff point beyond which elevated blood pressure is known to be more likely to cause complications.

Yet even if there is no sharp cutoff between traits and disorders, studies of extreme temperament (Rothbart, 2011) show how quantitative differences, at a given point, become qualitatively meaningful. An analogy offered by Kagan

(1989) is that in evolutionary theory, small differences between individual organisms eventually lead to the formation of new species.

We can apply the FFM to understand traits (Costa & Widiger, 2013). Extraverts are sociable, lively, and impulsive. Extraversion reflects individual differences in the need for interpersonal stimulation. This dimension is hypothesized to derive from baseline levels of arousal: introverts have a high level, which leads them to limit interpersonal contacts, while extraverts have a low level, which leads them to seek out more contacts. Variations in this trait do not necessarily correlate with psychopathology.

Neuroticism measures emotional stability. Individuals high on this dimension are easily upset, and take more time to calm down, while those low on this dimension are, using Galen's term, "sanguine". High neuroticism correlates with many mental disorders.

Agreeableness is an interpersonal construct related to emotional warmth versus coldness. Conscientiousness is related to behavioral control versus impulsivity. Low scores on both of these dimensions are related to PDs. However, the fifth of the five factors, openness to experience, has more to do with novelty seeking and creativity than with mental disorders.

Personality Is Heritable

A relatively new discipline, behavioral genetics (Knopik et al., 2016), has, over several decades, produced a large body of research that demonstrates the influence of genetic factors on personality. The most common method for determining the heritability of personality traits is by comparing their concordance in monozygotic (MZ) and dizygotic (DZ) twins. These studies show that for almost any broadly defined trait, MZ twins have a much higher concordance than DZ twins.

A statistical measure called heritability can be derived from this data. The finding that most personality traits have moderate to high heritability, usually in a range between 40% and 50%, has been frequently replicated, and studies that compare children who are adopted to their biological parents and to the parents who rear them yield similar estimates of heritability (Knopik et al., 2016).

The mechanisms by which genetic factors influence personality are complex. First, personality traits are influenced not by single genes but by the interaction of many genes (Rutter, 2006). Genome-wide association studies (GWAS; Sullivan, 2010) indicate that hundreds or thousands of polymorphisms can be correlated with mental disorders of all kinds, as well as with traits. Each genetic variation can also influence more than one type of behavior. Moreover, the true proportion of personality variance accounted for by genetic influence could be greater than 50%, since some of the residual variance involves interactive effects between genes and environment (Mitchell,

2018). For example, children directly influence the quality of their environment, by shaping the responses of others to conform to their traits (Scarr & McCartney, 1983).

Behavioral genetics also elucidates the importance of the environment. Even if the variance of most personality traits accounted for by genetic factors is close to 50%, there remains 50% to be accounted for by environmental factors. The most surprising findings of twin research concern the source of these influences. The environmental contribution to personality is largely *unshared*, i.e., not related to living in the same family (Knopik et al., 2016). Contrary to what one might expect, siblings growing up in the same family, like DZ twins, are hardly more similar in their personality than if they were perfect strangers.

The importance of the unshared environment could be explained in several ways. First, siblings may receive differential treatment from their parents. However, given that parents respond to a child's temperament, that could be just another example of gene–environment interactions. Second, variations in traits could lead individuals to perceive their environment differently. For this reason, retrospective data on childhood experiences can be shown to reflect heritable personality traits that influence memories of the past (Plomin & Bergeman, 1991). Third, experiences outside the family can be more important than what happens inside the family (Harris, 1998). While many experts have supported this idea, many remain incredulous that peers could be more important than parents in shaping personality. However, these relationships are not simple: research suggests that the unshared environment reflects, at least in part, gene–environment interactions (Mitchell, 2018). For example, children with temperamental vulnerabilities elicit more negative reactions. Yet the fact that adoption models give much the same result supports the conclusion that we need to place more emphasis on what is unshared.

The Minnesota Twin Study was the source of striking findings on the heritability of personality (Bouchard et al., 1990). This project used a design combining the advantages of twin and adoption studies by examining personality traits in MZ and DZ twins raised together and apart. Correlations between scores on a personality measure (the 11-dimensional Multidimensional Personality Questionnaire) for MZ twins were as high whether the twins were raised in the same family or separated at birth, while DZ twins had little concordance between personality traits.

An additional line of evidence supporting a genetic influence on personality traits is that broad personality dimensions are valid in cultures all over the world (Costa & Widiger, 2013). The effects of age in behavioral genetic studies of the variance in personality traits are even more affected by their genes. Some have suggested that people become "more like themselves" when they no longer live with their families of origin (Mitchell, 2018). Others note that personality becomes more stable with time, possibly because the environment has cumulative effects with aging (Briley & Tucker-Drob, 2014).

Personality Disorders Are Heritable

Are PDs as heritable as personality traits? In the previous edition of this book, I wrote that the evidence was insufficient to draw such a conclusion. However, we can now say that the answer is a definite yes.

While twin studies can have methodological limitations, all point in the same direction, showing that the heritability of most PDs is close to 50% (Torgersen, 2009). The best studies have come from Scandinavia. A twin sample in Norway (Torgersen et al., 2000) found that borderline personality disorder (BPD) was highly heritable, at 60%. In a larger sample of Cluster B disorders as defined by the *Diagnostic and Statistical Manual of Mental Disorders* (DSM), using a combination of interview and self-report measures, Torgersen et al. (2012) found the heritability of BPD to be 67%.

These findings are consistent with the view that most PDs are amplifications of heritable temperamental dispositions, measurable as traits. Even BPD, which is a more symptomatic disorder, has a heritability comparable to its underlying traits of affective instability and impulsivity.

We do not know how the heritability of personality traits and disorders translates into biological mechanisms. There are no biomarkers for any PD, and no genetic polymorphisms are specific to PDs as a whole, or to any category. Thus far, GWAS have been carried out only for BPD, and show that hundreds of genes, each with a small effect, can be involved (Witt et al., 2017).

Personality Traits Are Adaptations

The heritable factors in personality traits point to their having adaptive functions. This theory, that individual differences in traits represent alternative forms of adaptation, has been discussed by Beck and Freeman (2015).

One caveat must be registered: individual differences, whether in anatomy, physiology, or behavior, should not be assumed to be adaptive without specific empirical testing. Nevertheless, if traits are adaptations, this would explain a great deal about the functional significance of individual differences in personality. The hypothesis can be understood in the context of how organisms cope with an environment that is itself highly variable. Individual differences in personality would be alternate strategies, each of which could be more adaptive under one set of environmental circumstances, and less adaptive under another set of circumstances.

Let us consider two specific instances, each related to the clinical phenomena seen in patients with PDs. The first concerns the trait of shyness or "behavioral inhibition". This characteristic, operationally defined by a child's reaction to strangers, has long been known to have a strong genetic component (Kagan, 1994). Social avoidance could be adaptive under conditions where strangers present a real threat. In fact, through most of history, strangers *have* been dangerous, and continue to be so, in both large and small communities all over the world. The same trait would be maladaptive in a setting where threats from outsiders are rare, and in which shyness interferes with peer relationships, and even leads to social isolation.

A second example concerns impulsive traits. Impulsivity could reflect variability in autonomic activation affecting the timing of response to environmental challenges. Under conditions of immediate external danger, rapid responses are more adaptive. Impulsive traits become maladaptive when they continue to occur in the absence of real danger, and when they interfere with the development of rational judgments.

Why Personality Matters

Clinicians are mainly interested in symptoms for which they believe they have tools for treatment. For this reason, they often do not give enough priority to personality.

Yet research shows that most patients who have a PD do not respond to treatment in the same way as those who do not. Thus, antidepressants are often ineffective in the presence of a "comorbid" PD (Newton-Howes et al., 2006), and these agents are not recommended in the National Institute for Clinical Excellence (NICE) Guidelines for the treatment of BPD (NICE, 2009) or in the Cochrane reports (Stoffers et al., 2010).

When patients fail to respond to an antidepressant, clinicians often ignore personality factors and describe them as "treatment resistant" (Fava, 2003). This point of view underlies the practice of trying several different drugs, separately or together, for every patient with depressive symptoms. However, if a PD diagnosis is made, management can move in a different direction. We have good evidence that BPD can be treated with specialized forms of psychotherapy (Paris, 2010a). While these methods have not been adapted to manage other trait profiles, they may well be in the future.

Classifying Personality Disorders

The major obstacle to further progress in research on PDs is the absence of a reliable and valid system of classification. The history of science demonstrates that classifying phenomena is a precondition for the understanding of basic mechanisms. In biology, for example, without the detailed classification of organisms pioneered by Linnaeus, Darwin could have never developed an evolutionary theory. Unless we properly classify PDs, we cannot know what we are studying.

There are now multiple systems used for the classification of PDs. The *Diagnostic and Statistical Manual* (DSM-5; American Psychiatric Association, 2013) has two. One is the familiar 10-category list carried over from previous editions, which can be found in Section II of the manual. The other is an Alternative Model of Personality Disorder (AMPD), which uses dimensional assessment to create categories. This "hybrid" model can be found in Section III of DSM-5.

DSM-5, Section II, defines a PD as an enduring pattern of inner experience or behavior that deviates markedly from the expectations of the individual's culture, and manifests in at least two of the following sectors: cognition, affectivity, interpersonal functioning, or impulse control. In addition, the pattern must be inflexible or pervasive across a broad range of personal or social situations. It must lead to clinically significant distress or impairment in social, occupational, or other forms of functioning. Finally, the pattern must be stable and of long duration, with an onset that can be traced back to adolescence or early adulthood. There are 10 categories of PD, but a large proportion do not fit any of them and are therefore "unspecified".

The AMPD in Section III offers a different system. It defines a PD by levels of personality functioning: disturbances of self-functioning (identity and self-direction) as well as interpersonal functioning (empathy and intimacy). The AMPD also has criteria for maladaptive personality traits (negative affectivity, detachment, antagonism, disinhibition, and psychoticism). The next step involves assessment of pathological personality traits that are organized into five broad trait domains.

Note that DSM-5, in both models, no longer has an "Axis II". In previous editions, the use of a separate "axis" was designed to encourage clinicians to consider the diagnosis of PDs. However, this well-intentioned idea failed to achieve that goal, and the five-axis system was eliminated.

The *International Classification of Diseases* (ICD-11; World Health Organization, 2019) defines PDs in much the same way as DSM. However, it uses a different system that replaces categories with one based almost entirely on scoring personality traits and severity of dysfunction.

Clinicians are asked to score patients on five personality domains, as well as on functional impairment. Since many researchers on PD objected to the possibility of eliminating BPD, the ICD editors agreed to a compromise, and there is also a scoring option for a "borderline pattern", which resembles the criteria for BPD in DSM-5.

Comparing Categories and Dimensions

There is no universally accepted way to define PD categories. Psychiatrists are much in the same position as Linnaeus, who could only classify plants and animals by external appearance. In the absence of an etiological theory, they have had to base diagnosis on clinical phenomena.

The 10 categories of PD listed in DSM-5 Section II are "algorithmic", in that they use formal rules for diagnosis based on criteria sets. However, only two (borderline and antisocial) have attracted a large body of research. The

DSM categories were not based on systematic empirical data, but on clinical tradition. Some of the categories can be dropped, and the AMPD only recognizes six (schizotypal, antisocial, borderline, narcissistic, avoidant, and obsessive-compulsive).

In both DSM systems, many patients meet the general criteria for a PD, but not criteria for any of the specific categories. These "unspecified" cases constitute about half of the total (Zimmerman et al., 2005). That tells you all you need to know about the defects of these systems. However, the AMPD allows you to score their trait profile.

One problem is that medicine has a tradition of categorical diagnosis. DSM remains almost entirely categorical. The PDs in ICD-11 are a dimensional island in a categorical sea. While some have recommended dimensional diagnosis for all mental disorders (Kotov et al., 2017), psychiatry does not seem ready to adopt this idea.

Trait psychology evolved in a different way, preferring not to see PDs as separated from normal domains of personality, and as dimensions that can be scored quantitatively. The most important system arising from this tradition is the FFM (Costa & Widiger, 2013). Five domains of personality have been consistently found using factor analysis: openness to experience, conscientiousness, extraversion-introversion, agreeableness, and neuroticism. (The acronym "OCEAN" is helpful in remembering all five.) The domains are usually measured with self-report questionnaires (McCrae et al., 2005).

The FFM has been the subject of thousands of research papers. Yet it has not been adopted as a replacement for PD categories in psychiatry. The main reason is that it does a better job of describing normal personality variations than PDs.

Four of the five domains of the AMPD are similar to the FFM. Negative affectivity corresponds to neuroticism, detachment to introversion, antagonism to disagreeableness, and disinhibition to low conscientiousness. However, the fifth domain, psychoticism, does not parallel the construct of openness to experience.

The AMPD can be scored by clinicians, or by a self-report questionnaire, the Personality Inventory for DSM-5 (PID-5; Krueger et al., 2012). Two major advantages for the AMPD is that it allows for the construction of categories from the assessment of traits, and that it allows for description of trait profiles in patients who meet overall PD criteria but fall into an unspecified group.

The AMPD may eventually be adopted as the official DSM system, replacing the categories in Section II. The main reason this did not happen in 2013 was that the American Psychiatric Association felt that insufficient research was available to make a radical change. However, since then, the developers of the AMPD, especially Robert Krueger, have been highly energetic in conducting and promoting research on their model, and hundreds of papers have appeared in the literature.

The main limitation of the AMPD is that it is somewhat complicated to use. In a report on how clinicians view the system, it was seen as superior to Section II in several ways, although not in being more user-friendly (Morey et al., 2014).

ICD-11 goes much further in dimensionalizing PD diagnosis. It describes five trait domains (negative affectivity, detachment, dissocial, disinhibition, and anankastic) and has a five-level severity rating (Tyrer et al., 2011a). It is designed to be based on clinician ratings, but there are also ways to assess its constructs using self-report (Oltmanns & Widiger, 2019). The "borderline pattern", which does not fit this system, was pasted into the final version as an add-on to trait profiles.

There is one additional possibility, that mental disorders could eventually be diagnosed on the basis of changes in the brain, as in the Research Domain Criteria (RDoC; Insel et al., 2010). However, at this point, RDoC is not well rooted in empirical data, is relatively dismissive of the psychosocial factors in mental illness (Paris & Kirmayer, 2016), and has no system to account for the clinical phenomena seen in PDs.

In summary, diagnostic systems for PDs are in a state of flux, reflecting our lack of knowledge about the mental mechanisms behind these highly complex disorders. Yet in all fairness, hardly any of the diagnoses of symptomatic conditions in either DSM or ICD, including common and important entities such as depression, meet stringent criteria for diagnostic validity.

Personality disorder diagnoses are no different, and they remain syndromes, not true diseases. It is unlikely that we will soon develop a fully encompassing theory. The idea that we are ready to define mental disorders using neuroscience is premature and naïve. We will have to muddle along for many decades before we can reach that goal.

Personality Disorders Often Get Better with Time

It used to be thought that PDs are always chronic. However, that was only an example of a clinical bias (Cohen & Cohen, 1984) in which we continue to see the most severe cases of a disease, but no longer see milder cases that remit more readily, and do not request further treatment.

The large-scale Collaborative Longitudinal Personality Disorders Study (CLPS, Gunderson et al., 2011) followed a group of patients with four PDs (borderline, schizotypal, obsessive-compulsive, and avoidant) for 10 years to determine their outcome. The findings show that within two years, nearly half of cases no longer met criteria, largely due to reduction of symptoms, although functional levels did not improve much within this time frame.

A second study, focusing on BPD and a comparison group of other PDs, the McLean Study of Adult Development (MSAD; Zanarini et al., 2012) also found that patients improve over time and, importantly, that they rarely relapse. These findings, which are now based on a 24-year follow-up, confirm the results of earlier retrospective studies, and our own 27-year follow-back data showed that most BPD patients reach close-to-normal functioning by middle age (Paris, 2003).

These prospective design studies used in CLPS and MSAD have many advantages. However, since many patients do not sign up for such studies, retrospective data may help to provide a more generalizable picture of outcome. For example, in the MSAD study, the suicide rate for borderline PD patients is only 7%, but in several retrospective studies including more severely ill patients, the rate approached 10% (Paris, 2003). It is also notable that about 40% of BPD patients in the MSAD study remained dysfunctional after 24 years, even when they no longer had acute symptoms of the disorder.

Personality Disorders Are Treatable

Personality disorders do not respond well to antidepressants (Newton-Howes et al., 2006) or to mood stabilizers (Crawford et al., 2018). Even if some patients have a degree of symptomatic relief, their disorders do not remit when treated with any drug. On the other hand, we have striking evidence for the efficacy of specific methods of psychotherapy designed for BPD. The most studied method has been dialectical behavior therapy (DBT; Linehan, 1993), but several other methods have also been supported by clinical trials (Cristea et al., 2017). There is some evidence that psychological therapies can be effective within a few months (Laporte et al., 2018; McMain & Chapman, 2019).

It is notable that a large body of evidence shows that in psychological treatment, "common factors" are usually more important than specific techniques (Wampold, 2001). On the other hand, patients with moderate and severe PDs seem to require specific therapies that outperform nonspecific methods that have been called "treatment as usual" (Linehan, 1993).

Unfortunately, patients with PDs have problems accessing psychotherapy, which is expensive, as well as time- and resource-intensive. However, the good news is that the prognosis for most PDs is better than widely believed.

In summary, research showing that PDs tend to improve over time and are treatable should reduce the stigma attached to these diagnoses, and encourage clinicians to recognize them and to take on their treatment.

Chapter

Social Context and Personality

How to Assess Social Factors in Mental Disorders

Social psychiatry is concerned with the effects of social factors on the causes, course, and treatment of mental disorders. However, social risks are difficult to measure. There is no practical way to conduct controlled experiments in which their role can be isolated from other etiological factors. Research therefore uses indirect methods, so that conclusions inevitably require some degree of inference.

Two of the standard methods are prospective follow-up studies and case-control studies. In prospective studies, general community populations, or populations at risk, are followed over a number of years to see which individuals develop a disorder. These studies are relatively rare, but expensive and not always practical. Another problem is that cohorts followed over time tend to suffer from attrition.

Case-control studies compare patients who have already developed an illness to those without the disorder for the presence of risk factors. These studies are much more common. However, it is difficult to sort out which factors actually account for differences found between patient and nonpatient groups. Moreover, studies of patients do not examine risks in nonpatients.

For this reason, studies in the community tend to be better, since they can look for differences in prevalence in the general population, and measure relevant risk factors. Prevalence levels often vary with indicators that are related to social factors, such as demography, culture, or changes over time. If they do, one has presumptive evidence to suggest a role for social factors.

Socioeconomic class: One of the best known and most consistent findings in psychiatric epidemiology is a greater prevalence of major mental disorders in the lower socioeconomic classes (Dohrenwend & Dohrenwend, 1969). We can account for these social class differences in two contrasting ways. On the one hand, socioeconomic deprivation could be a risk factor for mental disorders (Hudson, 2005). On the other hand, belonging to a lower socioeconomic class could be the consequence of having a mental disorder. These two possible explanations have been called "origin versus drift", but both mechanisms are usually involved.

Cross-cultural differences: The presence of cross-cultural differences in prevalence provides convincing evidence for the role of social factors in mental disorders. It is possible that some of these differences could reflect biological variability. However, major mental disorders are found in all societies, albeit with somewhat variant symptoms (Murphy, 1982; Patel, 2001).

We can see the influence of culture most clearly in cases where the prevalence of a disorder has been low in a population, and then increases when its members emigrate to another society. An example is anorexia nervosa, which is rare in traditional societies, and can remain uncommon when families immigrate (Weissman, 2019). Anorexia has been increasing in Asian societies as they modernize (Pike & Dunne, 2015). Such findings provide strong evidence for the social shaping of psychopathology.

In a related scenario, historical changes convert underlying psychopathology into a different symptomatic form. One example is the shift from somatic presentations to psychological distress that Shorter (1992) described with the concept of a "symptom pool", in which culture determines the shape of overt psychopathology.

Cohort effects: Changes in prevalence over time offer the most powerful evidence for the presence of social factors in mental disorders. The increasing prevalence of a form of psychopathology in the same population over a single generation cannot be explained in any other way than social change. Researchers have documented cohort effects in several mental disorders (Keyes et al., 2014).

How Epidemiology Contributes to Understanding Psychopathology

Let us review some key findings concerning major categories of mental illness that have used epidemiological methods.

Schizophrenia: This condition is consistently more prevalent in lower socioeconomic groups. The weight of evidence suggests that this is largely due to drift, i.e., that schizophrenic patients move downwards in social class because of the social deterioration associated with their illness (Goldberg & Morrison, 1988; Hurst, 2007). While schizophrenia exists in all cultures, its severity varies, with more dysfunction in urban settings and industrialized countries (Murphy, 1982). Migrants from underdeveloped to developed societies often have a higher rate of the disorder (Cantor-Graae & Selten, 1995; Sharpley et al., 2001). However, this trend does not apply to all migrants, and varies greatly by country of origin (Morgan et al., 2019).

Depressive disorders: These conditions are also more common in lower socioeconomic classes (Freeman et al., 2016). Depression shows a notable difference in prevalence by gender, with rates two to three times higher among women (Weissman & Olfson, 1995). It has been a matter of some controversy whether this difference reflects genetic differences between the sexes, the effects of hormones, or differential social risk factors among females (Parker & Brotchie, 2010). It is also possible that the higher rate of substance use in men is a mirror image of depression, functioning as what psychiatrists used to call a "depressive equivalent".

The interacting effects of gender, social class, and psychological experiences were examined in a well-known study of the risk factors for depression in working class women in Britain (Brown & Harris, 1978). Depression was associated with specific psychological risk factors, such as the early loss of a mother, and the lack of a confiding relationship in adult life. However, this study also demonstrated the importance of social factors, as shown by higher rates of depression among women in working class London, as compared to women in a rural society (the Hebrides). These urban-rural differences in depression have also been found in other settings, including the USA (Robins & Regier, 1991). In a meta-analysis (Peen et al., 2010), most major mental disorders were found to be more common in cities. This suggests that urbanization can lead to social dislocation, raising the risk for psychopathology.

Even so, mental disorders are far from rare in rural settings. Srole and Fischer (1980) called the tendency to idealize rural life "the myth of paradise lost". There is a great deal of variability in the social integration of urban and rural life in different countries: cities in developing countries attract recent emigrants from rural areas. Rural societies in Europe traditionally tended to be village-based and tightly knit, while rural life in North America tended to isolate families.

Cross-cultural studies show that the clinical features of depression vary with culture. Guilt feelings and psychotic forms of depression are more common in Northern Europe and North America, whereas shame, somatic presentations, and paranoid symptoms tend to predominate in developing countries (Kleinman & Good, 1985).

North American studies have found a rising prevalence of depression in cohorts that have come of age in recent decades (Hidaka, 2012). This could reflect a real change, but it is also possible that it reflects a change in diagnostic practice following the popularity of antidepressant medication.

Alcohol use disorder: This condition has a higher prevalence in lower social classes (Grant, 1997). There is a striking gender difference, with male alcoholics outnumbering females by four to one, as well as major cross-cultural differences (Helzer & Canino, 1992).

Eating disorders: These conditions are convincing examples of the role of social factors in psychopathology. In the case of anorexia, modern culture supports the pursuit of thinness among young women (Gordon, 1990). Both anorexia and bulimia are rare in traditional societies. They therefore fall in a group of conditions that, unlike major psychiatric disorders, occur mainly in specific cultural contexts. These syndromes have therefore been called "culture-bound" (Prince & Tseng-Laroche, 1990).

The Prevalence of Personality Disorders

Epidemiology can also be applied to measure the prevalence of personality disorders in the general population. However, it runs into problems of measurement. Earlier studies did not examine PDs, and those that use trained assistants rather than experienced clinicians tended to overestimate prevalence. Most studies have found overall rates of PDs ranging between 10% and 13% (Coid et al., 2006; Lenzenweger et al., 2007; Torgersen et al., 2001). This may be an exaggerated estimate, given the lack of a clear boundary between personality and PD (Paris, 2010b).

The largest study of PD prevalence in the USA, the National Epidemiologic Survey on Alcohol and Related Conditions (NESARC; Grant et al., 2004) was originally designed to measure the prevalence of alcohol use disorder, but also yielded extensive data on PDs . Unfortunately, these findings are often quoted as definitive – which they are not, since they overestimated prevalence. Interviews were carried out in a community sample using trained raters, and scored with the Alcohol Use Disorder and Associated Disabilities Interview Schedule-5 (AUDADIS-5). The findings described a higher overall prevalence than all other studies. For example, borderline personality disorder (BPD) had a prevalence of nearly 6%, and the prevalence of obsessive-compulsive personality disorder (OCPD) was close to 8%. If you add up all the separate findings, you could get an overall PD prevalence of 21%. It is not inconceivable that one out of five have meaningful problems of some sort in work and relationships, but the conclusion that one out of five people have a PD is dubious. Again, these inflated levels reflect the difficulty of establishing a boundary between traits and disorders.

Another group of researchers went back to the data a few years later and set more rigid standards for diagnosis (Trull et al., 2010). Most differences in prevalence for individual diagnoses remained high, but were much lower than in the original study. Prevalence of any PD diagnosis decreased from 21.52% to 9.12%. The largest drops in rates occurred for schizoid (3.13%–0.57%), schizotypal (3.93%–0.62%), histrionic (1.84%–0.27%), narcissistic (6.18%–0.96%), and obsessive compulsive (7.88%–0.91%) personality disorders. BPD went down from 5.9% to 2.7%. Only antisocial personality disorder (ASPD) had a similar rate in the corrected data, at 3.8%.

Personality disorders also differ by gender. Antisocial personality disorder is much more common in males than in females (Black, 2015). Borderline personality disorder is as common in men in most epidemiological studies, but women dominate in clinical settings (Paris, 2015). Finally, PDs, like other mental disorders, have higher rates in urban populations and in lower socioeconomic groups, clustering in high-risk neighborhoods (Walsh et al., 2012).

Cohort Effects, Cross-Cultural Studies, and Historical Change

The best evidence for cohort effects on PDs is the increase in the prevalence of antisocial behavior after World War II, at the same time as rates of suicide and substance use also went up (Rutter & Smith, 1995). Indirect evidence suggests that these findings could also apply to BPD (Millon, 1993).

However, rates stabilized during the 1990s: crime, suicide, and even child abuse were reduced in prevalence (Finkelhor & Jones, 2006). In the subsequent years, the crime rate in the USA has continued to fall (Gramlich, 2019). The prevalence of child abuse has also continued to go down, although the frequency of childhood neglect remains stable (Charron, 1981). However, again in the USA, the frequency of suicidal ideation in women (Lövestad et al., 2019), suicidal attempts in both sexes (Olfson et al., 2017), and death by suicide in both men and women (Curtin et al., 2016) all went up again after 2000. The increase in death by suicide was most pronounced in middle-aged to older adults, but was also apparent in adolescents and young adults.

While these recent upward trends in suicide have been much discussed in the media, their meaning is unknown. What they demonstrate is the social sensitivity of suicide rates, which can vary in each decade and across national boundaries. However, we know that PDs are very frequent in young people who take their own lives (Lesage et al., 1994). Thus changes in suicide rates may therefore reflect changes in the prevalence of PDs, or changes in the extent to which PD leads to death. We also know that having a PD shortens the life span by at least a decade, even among those who do not die by suicide (Fok et al., 2014).

Unfortunately, historical or cross-cultural studies of PDs remain rare. One of the most striking findings in the literature was published 40 years ago, showing that even as antisocial PD became more common in Western countries, it remained rare in Taiwan (Hwu et al., 1989). This may or may not remain true today.

It is well known that mental disorders can present with different symptoms in different cultures, reflecting differences in the symptom bank (Gone & Kirmayer, 2010). However, it is less well known that symptoms can present differently in different historical periods (Shorter, 1997).

There are three ways in which historical changes in a culture can influence and shape the clinical presentation of psychopathology. The first concerns the choice of symptoms through which distress is expressed. At any given time, dysphoria can be communicated to others by an implicit choice from clinical presentations that are "out there" in the community, or in the symptom bank. The concept of "pathoplasty" (Jaspers, 1999; Mulder, 2004) describes the way that coexisting forms of psychopathology can shape observable clinical features.

A second mechanism involves social stressors that reduce thresholds for the development of psychopathology. While the symptoms of mental disorders derive from complex interactions between biological vulnerability, individual psychological experience, and sociocultural context, stressors can bring the interaction between risk factors to a tipping point at which distress causes overt symptomatology (Wexler, 2006).

A third mechanism concerns discrepancies between social demands and individual temperament in different historical periods and different social settings (Alarcón et al., 2009). To understand these relationships, we need to consider how social structures influence personality traits.

One mechanism behind this relationship is that behaviors that are acceptable in one culture may be seen as pathological in another (Alarcón et al., 1998). If the frequency of personality traits varies from one society to another, then the frequency of the disorders associated with trait dimensions should vary accordingly. Since PDs, by definition, describe a failure to meet social expectations, these conditions might be expected to show a higher degree of cultural sensitivity, i.e., responsiveness to variable sociocultural conditions (Paris, 2004).

Let us therefore examine to what extent social factors can shape personality traits, and the mechanisms by which social factors could lower the thresholds for traits to develop into disorders.

Society, Culture, and Personality Traits

The broad dimensions of personality are universal. Cross-national studies using the Five Factor Model (Costa & Widiger, 2013) have shown that similar personality traits can be found in all human societies. Variations in personality between individuals within a society can be greater than differences between one society and another. Yet these cross-cultural differences have an order of magnitude of about half a standard deviation (Eysenck, 1982).

Cross-cultural differences in personality could also reflect biological differences. Kagan (1994) reported that Chinese infants are temperamentally quieter and more inhibited than infants with Caucasian heredity. An alternate explanation of these differences is that societies shape personality traits through behavioral expectations. However, even if culture shapes personality, the extent of this influence may have been exaggerated. There is little evidence that each culture can be characterized by a modal personality structure. Instead, there are wide individual variations in personality within cultures (Costa & Widiger, 2013).

Even so, cultures value some forms of behavior more than others. By reinforcing or modeling different patterns of behavior, societies can reduce the frequency of traits that are contrary to social demands and increase the frequency of traits that are in accordance with social expectations. Essentially, culture increases the level of tolerance for some traits, and lowers the level for others.

Weisz et al. (1993) found that children brought up in traditional social structures tend to have more internalizing symptoms, while children raised in modern social structures are more likely to have externalizing symptoms. These findings are consistent with cross-cultural studies that found higher levels of extraversion and lower levels of neuroticism in modern societies than in traditional settings (Eysenck, 1982).

Emotional expressiveness is a good example of a personality trait that demonstrates cultural variability. Family therapists working with different ethnic groups have reported strong differences in how readily individuals communicated their feelings (McGoldrick et al., 1982). Families in traditional societies tend to encourage the repression of emotion more than those in modern societies (Eid & Diener, 2001). These differences reflect variations in how much societies value conformity to the group, as opposed to autonomy and individualism (Alarcón et al., 2009).

The mechanism by which culture shapes personality could involve transmission through the family, above and beyond genetic effects (Maccoby, 2000). Cultural values can also be transmitted through peer groups and social networks (Cavalli-Sforza et al., 1982). This is part of the mechanism by which socialization shapes personality (Harris, 1998), through peers, authority figures such as teachers, or through leaders of community organizations.

How do these mechanisms promote psychopathology? In general, social risk factors are structures characterized by normlessness, and by a lack of useful social roles (Leighton et al., 1963). Social protective factors would reflect structures characterized by clear norms and by adequate access to useful social roles.

Defined in this way, social risk factors are more common in modern societies, while social protective factors are more frequent in traditional societies. Thus PDs as a group could be less common in traditional societies. However, some personality profiles, such as extreme levels of impulsivity or social inhibition, would not fit well into any culture.

The Interface of Society and the Family

One of the main ways by which social structures influence the risk for psychopathology is through family functioning. Social disintegration makes family dysfunction more likely, and when family dysfunction is present, social risks amplify their effects. In contrast, social protective factors buffer the effects of family dysfunction.

The evidence that family dysfunction is one of the major psychological risk factors implicated in the etiology of the personality disorders is strong (Paris, 2015). However, families do not exist in isolation. It is entirely possible for families to be dysfunctional in a well-functioning society. If that pathology is sufficiently severe, children growing up in that family will be more likely to develop mental disorders, but social buffering could protect against this possibility. Conversely, even in the most dysfunctional society, well-functioning families can raise healthy children.

The social factors that most affect family functioning are the availability of supports for its members. These include employment opportunities, extended family, and community membership (Leighton et al., 1963). The absence of these supports is associated with an increased frequency of many forms of psychopathology. For example, any breakdown in the social environment, such as unemployment or the loss of support networks in the community could increase the prevalence of mental disorders. When the family loses support, parents become more dysphoric, lowering the quality of their care, and their children are more at risk.

One historian (Lasch, 1977) described the nuclear family in contemporary society as "a haven in a heartless world", but also saw it as "under siege". Modern families, as compared to families in traditional societies, are smaller and less stable. If the larger society fails to buffer the effects of family dysfunction, we have what medical researchers call a "double hit" mechanism. Modern nuclear families can more easily become overburdened. Geographical and social mobility uproots parents from extended families, as well as from the larger community. The resulting lack of outside support makes family breakdown more pathogenic. Yet while single risk factors can be more easily buffered, multiple insults can overwhelm defenses (Rutter, 2012).

It is fortunate that children suffering psychosocial disadvantages still show significant resilience. Thus the social environment buffers potentially damaging psychological experiences. Studies of "invulnerable" or "resilient" children point to social mechanisms that explain their relative lack of vulnerability (Werner & Smith, 1992). Resilient children have positive traits, can recognize pathology in their parents, and look elsewhere for attachments and models. In the larger society, there are many potential opportunities for alternate attachments. Good schools, as well as athletics and social clubs, have the potential to reduce psychopathology (Rutter & Rutter, 1993). These interfaces between attachments inside the family, and in the larger community, may be particularly important in contemporary life, in view of the changes in family structure that are occurring in every society, all over the world.

Cohort Effects and Risk Factors

Change in the frequency of mental disorders over a single generation cannot be biological. Cohort effects therefore point to social change.

The PD for which a cohort effect is best established is antisocial (Rutter & Smith, 1995), along with indirect evidence for an increase in the prevalence of BPD (Paris & Lis, 2013). The other categories have not been adequately studied. We do not know whether the prevalence of PDs as a whole is changing.

There are two possible explanations for cohort effects on the prevalence of PDs. The first involves changes in the frequency of risk factors associated with them. The second involves social change.

Family Breakdown

This risk factor stands out, and it has undergone a dramatic increase in frequency during the postwar era. In Western countries, about half of the children presently growing up in nuclear families will experience separation and divorce. This dramatic change has occurred over only the last few decades (Amato et al., 2009).

The long-term consequences of divorce for children are a good example of the principle that psychopathology develops only in the presence of multiple risk factors (Rutter & Rutter, 1993). However, family breakdown is likely to initiate a cascade of other negative consequences, which then provide the requisite multiple risks (Amato et al., 2009). After divorce, the custodial parent is often economically worse off, and the family is more likely to become geographically uprooted. In addition, the rate of divorce in second marriages is even higher than in first marriages (Riley, 1991). Finally, divorce is stressful for parents, and can make them psychologically less available (Wallerstein, 1989), leading to relative emotional neglect.

Severe parental conflict in an intact marriage can be at least as damaging as a parental separation (Rutter, 1971). This finding has sometimes been quoted to support the idea that effects of divorce can be positive. However, considering the mounting evidence that psychological complications more often follow from family dissolution, Rutter later stated that he had the responsibility to say that he was wrong (Rutter & Rutter, 1993).

Yet different types of family breakdown have different effects on children. Divorces that occur in the presence of parental mental disorders, or in situations of family violence, can have *relatively* positive outcomes, since children are relieved from being exposed to a traumatic environment (Hetherington et al., 1985). However, the majority of family breakdowns, which occur in the absence of either mental disorders or family violence, come as a disturbing and unpleasant surprise to children (Amato et al., 2009). Whatever the parental conflicts had been, they were not necessarily apparent to children who experience their intact family as positive and the breakdown of the family as negative (Wallerstein, 1989). Furthermore, one cannot make the bland assumption that even if a divorce can sometimes turn out to be positive for *parents*, it is a useful or even a neutral experience for *children*.

The best method of resolving questions about the impact of divorce is to follow children from the time of parental separation to adulthood. These studies (Hetherington et al., 1985; Wallerstein, 1989) have shown that the most severe sequelae of divorce are short-term, and that children tend to recover from these immediate effects. However, Wallerstein's cohort had many difficulties during late adolescence and young adulthood. They were less likely to attain an educational level consonant with their economic background, found it more difficult to decide on a career, and had more problems in establishing stable relationships.

What research on the outcome of divorce has not addressed is whether family breakdown has a differential effect on vulnerable populations. Most children of divorce are probably resilient enough to develop normally. This might not be the case for those with diatheses to mental disorders, such as extreme temperaments. Separation or loss may be more likely to lead to psychopathology in children with trait vulnerabilities. These interactions between temperament and experience have not yet been studied.

In summary, in looking for a social risk factor that could account for cohort effects on the prevalence of PDs in modern societies, the increased rate of family breakdown is a strong candidate. Although we lack firm evidence at present to support this general hypothesis, there is an association between family breakdown and disorders in the impulsive cluster (Paris, 2020).

Even so, family breakdown by itself is neither necessary nor sufficient for the development of PDs. Like all the other psychological variables, it is not a cause, but a *risk factor* for psychopathology. This means that while it could make the development of a PD more likely, many individuals with such disorders come from intact families. It also means that a cumulative risk is probably only meaningful when combined with biological factors, with other psychological risks, and with the impact of social factors.

It is possible that research into the effects of divorce and single parenting may have been inhibited by the contemporary social climate, which is either tolerant of or favorable to divorce, and which assumes that traditional family structures are outmoded and can be replaced by alternate arrangements. The empirical literature reviewed above can be interpreted as supporting the idea that a two-parent nuclear family, whatever its inherent problems, is, by and large, a better environment for children than other alternatives. The position taken here is that there is sufficient evidence for social psychiatrists to support the importance of "family values".

Emotional Neglect

In theory, two mechanisms might lead to increased emotional neglect of children in modern society. The first involves a geographical and social uprooting of nuclear families: when parents receive less support, they may provide less care to their offspring. The second concerns changes in social values: narcissism in parents might lead them to be less interested in their children.

However, there is, in fact, *no* evidence that children are receiving a lower quality of parenting in modern society. If anything, the historical evidence suggests that parents in the past probably had *less* interest in the lives of their children (deMause, 1974). Current problems in parenting may be more related to overprotection than to neglect (Twenge, 2011).

Trauma

Are traumatic experiences during childhood increasing in frequency in modern society? One might imagine, for example, that as the frequency of family breakdown increases, more children are being raised by step-parents, who are more likely than biological parents to be involved in either the sexual abuse (Browne & Finkelhor, 1986) or the physical abuse of children (Malinovsky-Rummell & Hansen, 1993).

Again, there is *no* evidence that child abuse is becoming more common. On the contrary it is clearly decreasing (Finkelhor et al., 2005, 2013, 2014). Thus while traumatic childhood experiences may be more *apparent* than they once were, they are not more common than they were 50 years ago.

Parental Psychopathology

If parental psychopathology has been increasing the risk for the development of PDs is becoming more frequent, this could also have an effect on prevalence. There have indeed been marked cohort increases in depression (Hidaka, 2012) and in substance abuse (Degenhardt et al., 2016) in the generations that are now raising children. Since these disorders are more likely to be associated with family breakdown, cohort effects on risk factors might involve interactions between a higher prevalence of parental psychopathology and an increased rate of parental separation. However, there is no evidence to support this hypothesis.

In conclusion, the presence of a social risk factor *by itself* is generally insufficient to produce a PD. Risk factors have their greatest effect on children who are already vulnerable by virtue of their personality traits. Most likely, a pathological social environment *amplifies* the effects of biological and psychological risk factors.

Chapter

Modernity and Personality Disorder

Traditional and Modern Societies

Social structures can be broadly dichotomized into "traditional" or "modern" types (Giddens, 1991; Inkeles & Smith, 1974). Traditional societies are primarily characterized by slow rates of social change, and by intergenerational continuity. Modern societies, in contrast, are characterized by rapid social change, and by intergenerational discontinuity. This dichotomy tells us something useful about the evolution of culture.

However, societies are constantly changing, and there are important differences between the traditions of all societies that could be classified as "traditional". Whatever their specific nature, these structures provide individuals with a set of predictable expectations. For this reason, traditional structures have the potential to buffer psychopathologies related to behavioral dyscontrol.

The 19th-century German sociologist Ferdinand Tonnies (1974) described modernity as a shift from "gemeinschaft" (rewards based on group membership) to "gesellschaft" (rewards based on productivity). Another way of looking at this dichotomy between traditional and modern societies is to describe cultures as *collectivist* or *individualistic* (Markus & Kitayama, 1991). In traditional societies, identity is bound to the family and to the larger values of society. In modern societies, identity is unique to the individual and has to be created de novo.

The breakdown of stable structures, and their replacement by less stable ones, as has been occurring in modern societies, creates *rapid social change*. Instability in the social fabric can be a risk factor for psychopathology in general (Asmolov, 2016) and for personality disorders (PDs) in particular (Paris, 2015).

Not all PDs are associated with social change. The structures of traditional societies tend to favor personality traits that sometimes carry risks of their own. These societies have less tolerance for deviance, and tend to "outgroup" individuals whose traits or behaviors fail to meet their expectations. In some traditional societies that have been studied by anthropologists, people with antisocial behaviors may even be killed off (Chagnon, 1988).

For most of its members, traditional societies provide relatively secure and predictable roles for every individual. There is a price to pay, however. To make conformity with family and community expectations normative, these social structures tend to promote emotional and behavioral inhibition (Asmolov, 2016). By contrast, modern societies demand a high level of autonomy. Here there is a different price to pay. People are expected to create their own roles, even if doing so is not easy. The result is that many people in modern societies are afflicted by loneliness and unemployment (Putnam, 2000).

Social Integration and Social Disintegration

In a classical research project on social factors in mental disorders, the "Stirling County Study" (Leighton et al., 1963) compared two Nova Scotia communities that varied in levels of what the authors called "social integration". One of these communities was relatively well integrated, whereas the other was not. The level of social integration in each setting was measured by an index that was an amalgam of many factors, including broken homes, absence of social associations, weak leadership, few patterns of recreation, frequent crime, poverty, cultural confusion, secularization, migration, and social change.

The main finding was that there was a higher level of psychopathology in the less integrated community. The authors hypothesized that sociocultural disintegration fosters psychiatric disorders by interfering with physical security, by being more permissive in the expression of sexual and aggressive impulses, by interfering with intimate relationships and economic success, as well as with finding a place in society, in a group, or in a moral order.

In many ways, the theoretical principles used by the Stirling County study resemble those proposed by the French sociologist Emil Durkheim (1897/1997) to account for changes in the prevalence of suicide. Durkheim observed the varying rates in European societies over time, and evolved a construct he called "anomie", or normlessness. Similarly, the theory of social integration–disintegration predicts that societies that are more integrated, i.e., those with clear norms, protect individuals from psychopathology, while in those with weak norms psychopathology will be more likely.

Research continues to support anomie as an explanation for variations in suicide rates. However, research has consistently shown that happiness is not correlated with economic growth (Easterlin, 2015). In a study of differential prevalence of suicide across Canadian provinces carried out over 30 years ago, Zakinofsky and Roberts (1987) found that the highest rates occurred in regions with the most economic development. This seeming paradox makes more sense if one considers that rapid development breaks down traditional values. In the Canadian study, suicide was most frequent among those who were left behind by progress, i.e., the unemployed men. In more traditional provinces, such as Newfoundland, the suicide rate remained low in spite of much higher levels of unemployment. In Québec, where cultural traditions have been strong, a governmental study from the same period (Charron, 1981) found that suicide rates were highest in mining communities, where people had few roots, and lowest in traditional rural communities or towns where people had a sense of cultural continuity.

Durkheim's concept of anomie, which parallels the construct of social disintegration, is crucial. It is particularly important in accounting for high suicide rates found in indigenous populations, particularly affecting young males (Kirmayer et al., 2000). The breakdown of a traditional way of life often means that young people are unable to establish social roles. Again, those who are already vulnerable because of both personality traits and negative family experiences are more susceptible to the effects of a pathological social environment.

These mechanisms help to explain cohort effects on the prevalence of psychopathology. As described in Chapter 3, there has been an increase in Western countries of problems associated with emotional dysregulation (including depression, parasuicide, and completed suicide) and with impulsivity (substance abuse and criminality). These problems could be due to the relative absence of secure attachments in contemporary society (Linehan, 1993).

The vicious circle here is that breakdown of traditional social structures is associated with a breakdown of family structures. The dissolution of families is one of the defining features of social disintegration, and tends to be a consequence of social pathology. When nuclear families are isolated from the community, they lose stability due to lack of extrafamilial support, as has been shown in research on the risks for divorce (Amato et al., 2009). Moreover, children from broken families, who might more readily find alternative attachments and models in a more integrated society, will be less able to do so, leading to social isolation and/or bonding with pathological peer groups (Millon, 1993).

Social Change and Modernity

Culture normally changes in a gradual fashion, through quasi-evolutionary mechanisms (Durham, 1992). The breakdown of norms associated with rapid social change interferes with this process. During the course of human history, most social norms have been traditional, but today most societies have adopted modernity. Richerson and Boyd (2006) developed models of interactions between biology and culture that make relying on tradition more advantageous as compared to constant experiment. When social change is gradual, it is easier for individuals to adapt and to create new social roles.

"Modernity" describes the social and cultural conditions that characterized the 20th century (Taylor, 1992). Modern societies have led to many valuable developments and offer a wider range of social opportunities. Most people, and women in particular, have benefited from progress and the freedom to develop new ideas. Very few would want to live in any other type of society. However, there are important trade-offs.

What is unique in modern society is the continuous *acceleration* of social change. It has irreversibly changed traditional societies all over the globe, leading to smaller family size, higher geographic and social mobility, and a fragmentation of social norms (Giddens, 1991). Thus modernity replaces predictable expectations with choices. In modern society, each individual has to create personal norms. When the rate of social change is sufficiently high, the norms for role performance that were valid for an older generation are no longer useful. Young people face a particularly stressful task, in having to forge a personal identity, sometimes without access to role models. Young men are most at risk, as shown by higher suicide rates (Kirmayer et al., 2000).

It may be useful to apply Erikson's (1950) concept that the developmental task of adolescence is identity formation. However, the idea that each generation must forge its identity is a new development in history. In traditional societies, the family and community, not the individual, were responsible for choices of work, partners, and community affiliations. In such societies, *not* allowing the young to choose psychosocial roles assured intergenerational continuity.

In spite of rapid social change, most young adults successfully manage to develop both personal identity and social roles. Yet the process of identity formation demands a capacity for individuation for autonomy. The most autonomous individuals are those who have positive personality trait profiles and have had secure bonds in their families (Belsky & Cassidy, 1994). The loss of intergenerational continuity is most stressful for young people who lack these advantages.

The problem of identity lies on an interface between society and the family. In order to develop a personal identity, young adults need both family and social supports. Rapid social change makes the transmission of values from parents to children more difficult. At the same time, the nuclear family is becoming more unstable. The children of divorce are somewhat more likely to flounder during young adulthood if they lack a secure base for attachment and parental guidance (Wallerstein, 1989). The divorce "epidemic" is itself a reflection of a society that values individualism more than loyalty to the group, and which therefore sees dissolving a family as legitimate as long as it benefits the member who leaves (Amato et al., 2009).

Because disintegrated or anomic societies are radically individualistic, they may fail to provide a sense of meaning and belonging for young people. Modern society demands adaptation to a number of new challenges, including an increased life span, a decrease in family size, changes in family structure, new conditions of work, and ideological confusion (Westen, 1985). These trends have been described by Twenge and Campbell (2009) as promoting narcissism in young adults.

Changes in society in very recent years have also been hypothesized to be problematic for young people. Lukianoff and Haidt (2019) point to increases in overprotective parenting and the decline of activities such as autonomous play, as failing to prepare adolescents for adult functioning. Twenge et al. (2017) note that the near universal use of smartphones has had various negative consequences, including interference with normal sleep, decreases in face-to face interactions, as well as exposure to toxic social comparison and bullying. While other large-scale surveys suggest that these effects are relatively small (Orben et al., 2019), they may still be clinically important if they have effects on adolescents who are temperamentally vulnerable.

In targeting aspects of modernity as risk factors, we need not idealize past societies, which had their own share of both social and family pathology, nor should we ignore the social tensions in existing traditional ones. Every generation is tempted to believe that life was better in the past. There is a real danger of "cultural nostalgia", in which we imagine either the previous state of our own society or that of other societies as "lost Edens" (Srole & Fischer, 1980). We should view the effects of modernization in the context of the ubiquity of social tension and conflict.

Modernity and Personality Disorders

Personality disorders develop out of discordances between trait variations and social expectations. The same traits can be adaptive or maladaptive in different societies, depending on whether they have a traditional or a modern structure. Chapters 5–8 will provide examples of these relationships.

The overall principle is that modern society values some personality trait profiles but not others. It favors individualism, celebrating those who are most accomplished in their work, not those who value attachments to other people. These traits tend to be adaptive in societies that value autonomy. It is only when they are highly amplified (as in antisocial or narcissistic PD) that they lead to major problems. However, as we will see in Chapter 7, these traits are becoming more common in modern societies.

Traditional societies have an opposite response to many of the same traits. These societies value group cohesion above all, and rein in those who are too self-centered. In a traditional society, one is expected to show strong deference to elders in any decision process and to be cautious with strangers outside the family. Such societies may therefore value dependence, which increases group cohesion, as well as avoidance, which makes it more likely that individuals will remain attached to their families. People who lack social skills may fare better in traditional societies that can provide socially undemanding employment and that can arrange marriages. This social buffering makes it less likely that individuals with these traits will develop certain types of personality disorder.

Moreover, family and social structures can contain impulsive personality traits, which is less likely in modern societies.

As long as traits remain adaptive, there is room in any society for variety on personality. Stone (1993) suggested that stable societies have an "ecological" balance among traits, and that this balance breaks down in rapidly changing societies. When a society undergoes a transition from tradition to modernity, some personality characteristics can become maladaptive. Social and historical transitions are therefore times of particular risk for the development of PDs.

In summary, modernity makes psychological development more difficult for some but easier for others. Modern societies benefit those who can achieve a high level of autonomy, but there are many who are not able to cope with this expectation. These demands function as a social "selection pressure". Some will benefit, and the effects of social change can be neutral for the majority, but in a vulnerable minority, they can lead to psychopathology.

Chapter

5

The Borderline Pattern

An Overview of Borderline Personality Disorder

Borderline personality disorder (BPD) is common, both in the community and in the clinic. Nevertheless, this condition has had an uphill battle to be recognized, and the diagnosis remains controversial. In accord with the *International Classification of Diseases* (ICD-11; World Health Organization (WHO), 2019), the title of this chapter uses its term: a *borderline pattern*. However, I will make the reader's life easier by referring to BPD.

Borderline personality disorder is a syndrome, and not in the full medical sense a disease. However, it is no less valid than most of the diagnoses in the *Diagnostic and Statistical Manual of Mental Disorders* (DSM) system, which is more widely used than ICD-11. It seems likely that the description of BPD in DSM-5, either the traditional one in Section II, or the alternative system in Section III, will continue to dominate research and practice for years to come.

Borderline personality disorder has suffered from its reputation as an obscure derivative of psychoanalytic theory. Stern (1938) was the first to describe patients who function on a "border" between neurosis and psychosis. More descriptive terms would have been better, such as "emotionally unstable personality disorder" or "emotion regulation disorder", which at least describe the characteristic psychopathology of the condition. For now, we are stuck with a misnomer.

The definition of BPD in DSM-5, Section II, requires the presence of at least five of nine criteria: fear of abandonment, intense unstable relationships, identity disturbance, impulsivity, recurrent suicidal behavior, affective instability, emptiness, inappropriate anger, and transient paranoid ideation or dissociative symptoms. The Alternate Model of Personality Disorders (AMPD) system in DSM-5, Section III, builds the BPD diagnosis from a trait profile, which is a more complex procedure, but one that yields a similar profile. The ICD-11 definition of a borderline pattern is very similar.

Gunderson and Singer (1975) were the first to show that BPD was a construct that could be operationalized, and in the ensuing years, the disorder became the subject of an extensive empirical literature (Paris, 2020). There are now over 3,000 papers on BPD listed on Medline.

Borderline personality disorder may vary across national boundaries, but it is not a culture-bound syndrome. It was the most frequent PD diagnosis among clinical populations in a WHO cross-national study (Loranger et al., 1994). It has been shown to be commonly recognizable in clinical populations of suicide attempters in India (Pinto et al., 2000), in China (Zhong & Leung, 2007), and in Turkey (Senol et al., 1997).

The most relevant data comes from a WHO survey conducted in 13 countries (Huang et al., 2009). The results showed that 1%–2% of people in most of these countries studied met criteria for a "Cluster B" PD (i.e., a group of diagnoses defined by DSM-IV and characterized by impulsive behavior patterns). Cluster B diagnoses were more common in the young, but cross-national differences were inconsistent, possibly reflecting sampling variation. Unfortunately, BPD was not examined separately, and these results are difficult to generalize because Cluster B also includes the more prevalent category of dissocial (antisocial) personality disorder. However, even if these methods did not allow for a test of cross-cultural difference in prevalence, the survey shows that this group of disorders is common around the world.

Borderline personality disorder patients have a wide range of culture-specific impulsive behaviors that fall within the broader category of *externalizing* disorders. As discussed in Chapter 4, these problems are more frequent in developed countries. This is why BPD is probably less common in non-Western than in Western societies.

Borderline personality disorder has a community prevalence of about 1%–2%, both in the USA (Lenzenweger et al., 2007; Trull et al., 2010) and the UK (Coid et al., 2006). Since BPD patients are help-seeking, the clinical prevalence is higher, affecting about 9% of all outpatients (Zimmerman et al., 2005). About half of all patients coming to emergency rooms with recurrent suicide attempts meet criteria for this diagnosis (Forman et al., 2004).

Although many cases of BPD can be typical, the diagnosis, like most categories in psychiatry, is fuzzy around the edges. Tyrer (2009) criticized the construct on these grounds; i.e., that patients meeting criteria can be quite heterogeneous. He is right, but that is also true of every category in the DSM-5 and ICD-11. It remains clinically important to identify BPD, because it requires entirely different treatment from the conditions with which it has a family resemblance (major depression and bipolar disorder). Psychiatrists in emergency rooms are familiar with patients who present with either over-doses, or wrist slashing, usually following a conflict in an intimate relationship.

The key clinical feature that underlies BPD is emotional dysregulation or affective instability (Linehan, 1993). Zimmerman et al. (2019) have shown that this one criterion, by itself, can be used as a screen for BPD. The abnormal mood in BPD is quite unlike the stable depression seen in classical mood disorders. In contrast to states of depression, mood is highly reactive and responsive to environmental factors (Gunderson & Phillips, 1991). Patients often describe their emotions as being "on a roller coaster".

The gender distribution of BPD in clinical settings is about 80% female (Zimmerman et al., 2005). Interestingly, community studies, including a British report (Coid et al., 2006), as well as an American study, the large-scale National Epidemiologic Survey on Alcohol and Related Conditions (Grant et al., 2004), have found the disorder to be equally common in males. However, males with BPD are less likely to be help-seeking. (As I tell my students, men don't like to ask for directions.)

Borderline personality disorder is too complex to be accounted for either by the present state of knowledge in the neurosciences, or by adverse life experiences. A combination of multiple factors carries most of the risk.

Twin studies indicate that at least half the variance in BPD is heritable (Reichborn-Kjennerud et al., 2013). However, no specific polymorphism is linked to the disorder, and genome-wide association studies (GWAS) find that hundreds of genes, each with a small effect, can be identified (Witt et al., 2017). There are also no biological markers specific to BPD, and it is not strictly an endophenotype.

Cross-sectional retrospective studies, as well as prospective studies, point to the psychological factors associated with BPD. The risks include traumatic experiences, such as childhood sexual and/or physical abuse, but only about a third of patients have such histories, and the most consistent childhood adversity in BPD is emotional neglect (Paris, 2020). This is more or less the same as what Linehan (1993) called "invalidation". In other words, BPD patients cannot manage strong emotions, and lack access to people who understand how they feel. This is a good example of a gene–environment interaction.

The symptoms of BPD do not last indefinitely, but tend to "burn out" in middle age (Paris, 2003). While between 5% and 10% eventually commit suicide, most do not. By age 40, the majority will no longer meet criteria for the diagnosis. The mechanisms for recovery over time could involve both biological maturation and gradual social learning. This having been said, patients may have fewer active symptoms over time but do not always achieve stable psychosocial functioning (Zanarini, 2005).

Borderline personality disorder used to be considered untreatable, but we now have a number of evidence-based psychotherapies for these patients. The best known, and the most widely researched, is dialectical behavior therapy (DBT; Linehan, 1993). This method targets the problem of emotion dysregu-lation: when patients learn to identify and manage emotions, and not to act on them impulsively, they usually improve in other ways.

Borderline Personality Disorder in Historical Context

Prior to the pioneering paper by Stern (1938), which described BPD in a recognizable way for modern clinicians, there were no published descriptions of the disorder or even of such characteristic features as self-harm. Borderline personality disorder only became the basis of formal diagnosis in the latter half of the 20th century (Berrios, 1993; Stone, 1997). One does not have to go far in the historical literature to find descriptions of psychosis or severe depression. In contrast, it is difficult to find historical evidence that typical BPD symptoms such as chronic self-harm or repetitive suicidal behaviors were common 100 years ago. It is possible that this clinical picture is a relatively recent development. If so, social risk factors would have to be invoked to account for the change.

On the other hand, the *traits* underlying BPD could have been just as prevalent in the past. As shown by cross-cultural studies, personality dimensions do not show large cross-cultural differences (McCrae & Costa, 1997), even if the symptoms associated with them vary. It is also possible that some of these problems were not medicalized and/or not recognized.

In the course of history, some people have always attempted suicide. Yet there are no reports in the older medical literature, or descriptions in the historical literature, of a pattern of mood instability, recurrent overdoses or self-harm, and unstable relationships. In fact, deliberate self-harm, in the form of superficial cutting of the wrist, was first described in the literature a little more than 50 years ago (Graff & Mallin, 1967; Pao, 1967). While some religious rituals are associated with cutting (Favazza, 1987), such behaviors have an entirely different motivation.

The underlying trait vulnerabilities behind BPD, affective instability and impulsivity (Crowell et al., 2009), can find expression in other ways. When societies modernize, one can see changes that Shorter (1992) called a "symptom pool", so that one set of symptoms is replaced by another. Abnormal mood could have presented primarily with somatic symptoms in the past. In most parts of the world, distress is more likely to be expressed somatically. So-called hysterical or conversion symptoms were one of the concerns of 19th-century psychiatry, but have become rare in Western societies (Merskey, 1997), but remain common in traditional societies (Littlewood, 2002). These physical symptoms can be understood as functioning to mobilize family and community to deal with mental distress (Kirmayer & Young, 1998).

A study from rural India (Nandi et al., 1992), illustrates the point. Researchers had found a high frequency of conversion symptoms when a primary care population was first surveyed, but when they returned to the same site 15 years later, these symptoms had become rare, while overdoses became much more common. In a kind of historical "fast forward", this sequence could reflect changes that have already occurred in the symptom pool of Western society over the last century. Thus, when the main form of expression for distress was somatic, physicians diagnosed patients with conversion and "neurasthenia". This was also the case for Chinese society, at least until relatively recently (Prince & Tseng-Laroche, 1990). Today, impulsive symptoms have become a more common way for emotional distress to be expressed.

The concept of a "symptom pool" describes that while psychological distress occurs at all times and all places, at any given historical moment or social context, the environment shapes symptoms by offering specific symptomatic options to express distress. The concept goes beyond the familiar cultural coloring of psychopathology, as in the specific content of psychotic delusions. Instead, diagnoses in entirely different groups can be transformed by social influences (Shorter, 1992).

This paradigm is further reinforced by the construct of *social contagion*, in which symptoms are spread either through personal contact or through the media (Rodgers et al., 1998). These mechanisms correspond to what Dawkins (1976) and Blackmore (1999) term *memes*. Clinical studies suggest that patients can learn about self-harm behaviors through social contagion, learning about wrist-cutting from peers and from media reports (Nixon & Heath, 2008). For example, it has been observed that patients without a history of self-harm admitted to a hospital ward alongside self-harming patients sometimes begin to cut themselves (Taiminen et al., 1998). In current times, influenced by the power of the Internet, there are new ways for patients to learn how to harm themselves. They can learn these techniques by looking them up on YouTube.

In summary, BPD is a disorder that could be of relatively new historical onset, and that has been described most often in Westernized societies. Its specific symptoms can be spread through social contagion, and the culture's symptom bank contains the signs and symptoms clinicians know and look for. It is also possible that people in developing societies are less likely to somatize, and more likely to express distress by self-harm and suicidal attempts.

Social Risk Factors in Borderline Personality Disorder

The social risk factors in BPD have not been the subject of much research. However, indirect, but converging, evidence suggests that BPD is increasing in prevalence in North America and Western Europe. This conclusion can be based on studies of its most common behavioral symptoms. An example is the dramatic increase in the youth suicide rate over the 1960s to 1990s (Rutter & Smith, 1995). In a Canadian sample, using a method called "psychological autopsy", about a third of youth suicides were retrospectively diagnosed as having had BPD (Lesage et al., 1994). This trend also applies to the frequency of suicide attempts over the same period (Bland et al., 1998). Moreover, these increases apply to self-harm, both in the USA, with a tripling of the rate over

15 years (Mercado et al., 2017) and in the UK, with a 68% increase over a similar period (Morgan et al., 2017).

These changes overlap with the development of new platforms for *social contagion*, a mechanism for spreading symptoms in the population. One could be increased screen time on social media (Lukianoff & Haidt, 2019; Twenge et al., 2017). These authors note that changes in rates of depression in adolescence increased at the same time as smartphones became universal. A recent meta-analysis of the empirical literature (Keles et al., 2019) supported a relationship between exposure to social media and significant increases in depression and self-harm in adolescent girls (who are more vulnerable to social exclusion). However, one cannot be sure that these correlations are causal, since longitudinal cohort studies would need to be conducted.

At the same time, the risk factor that some studies have found to be strongly associated with BPD, child abuse, is becoming *less* frequent (Finkelhor et al., 2013). Today's parents are more aware of dangers, and do not allow their children to be alone to the same extent as in past generations. Nevertheless, there is no evidence that BPD is becoming less common. (If it seems to be more common, that is probably because more clinicians are familiar with the construct and willing to make the diagnosis.)

It still remains possible that borderline personality disorder, rarely if ever described before1938, may have increased in prevalence since then. If so, that could reflect the effects of social forces, specifically the problems of modernity. This was the basis of Millon's (1993) model of the role of social factors in BPD. Applying social learning theory and the concept of anomie (Durkheim, 1897/1997), he argued that a loss of meaning and the social disintegration that characterizes contemporary society has a particularly negative effect on youth. A breakdown of social norms and rapid social change can interfere with the intergenerational transmission of values, reducing the influence of family and community. Thus, modern social communities would be more fragile, failing to buffer and compensate for defects in parenting.

Determining the influence of culture on psychiatric disorders requires data from epidemiological studies. Unfortunately, the community prevalence of BPD in less developed countries is unknown. The WHO survey conducted in 13 countries (Huang et al., 2009) found that 1%–2% of people around the world meet criteria for a "Cluster B" PD, and these diagnoses were most common in the young. However, cross-national differences were inconsistent, possibly reflecting sampling variation, and BPD was not examined separately.

Borderline personality disorder may nonetheless be less common in non-Western than in Western societies, in part due to the fact that impulsive behaviors are culture-specific, and in part to the stresses of modernity. Thus *externalizing* disorders – as opposed to *internalizing* disorders, in which suffering is expressed through inner distress rather than through impulsive behaviors (Achenbach & McConaughy, 1997) – is a factor analytically defined dimension that cuts across many diagnoses in psychiatry (Eaton et al., 2010; Krueger et al., 2011). This construct includes behaviors such as criminality, substance abuse, bulimia nervosa, and suicide attempts. These are the same problems that have increased in prevalence over recent decades.

Borderline personality disorder is a complex construct that also shows features of internalizing disorders. Borderline personality disorder patients are high in the personality trait of neuroticism (Costa & Widiger, 2013). Thus, the self-harm behavior often seen in these patients can be understood both as an impulsive action and as a way of regulating dysphoria (Brown et al., 2002).

One could draw implications for prevention from this data. People who eventually develop BPD may need more than average help in controlling their emotions and the impulsive actions linked to emotion dysregulation. Because these patients are thin-skinned, they do not easily brush off minor conflicts and rejections. This problem could be buffered by a supportive family that provides validation for negative emotions. However, not all families are like that. Even in this age of "helicopter parenting", some people advise their children to bear up sorrows and move on. This strategy may work well for children who are emotionally insensitive, but in those who are overly sensitive to their environment (Rioux et al., 2018), the result can be a build-up of dysregulation that explodes in adolescence.

Children do not only depend on their parents for emotional support and connection, and peer groups are of at least equal importance (Millon, 1993), but sensitive children have more trouble making the kind of friends they need. They are often too different for their peers to accept, and can become socially isolated and/or bullied. For this reason, the social environment often fails to provide support that was missing from the family.

Theorists attempting to account for BPD have also proposed that modern society makes the modulation of dysphoric affects more difficult, due to a relative absence of consistent social support (Linehan, 1993). These risks have increased with rapid social change, in spite of the unprecedented affluence of modern society.

Another line of evidence comes from clinical observations suggesting that patients who have not suffered from BPD in their country of origin can develop this condition once they immigrate to the West (Paris, 1996). One possible explanation is that when one grows up in a more traditional society, behavior is more closely monitored, and emotional stability is promoted by having provided social roles, associated with the support of extended families and a tightly knit community.

The mechanisms by which social factors affect the risk for BPD could also depend on "social sensitivity", a construct that describes the likelihood that individuals will respond symptomatically to social change (Paris, 2004). Many socially sensitive disorders (e.g., substance abuse, eating disorders, antisocial personality, borderline personality) have prominent externalizing symptoms that are particularly responsive to social context.

Another clue to the role of social factors in BPD is that this condition, as well as other externalizing disorders, begins in adolescence, a developmental stage that can be stressful, at least for some. Adolescence is in part a social construction (Furstenberg, 2000), since throughout most of history, young people assumed adult roles earlier in life. However, in a modern society, where adolescents have to find their own path, this stage can be stressful, particularly for those who are temperamentally vulnerable (Paris, 1997). Thus young people who are at risk because of temperamental vulnerability and exposure to psychological adversity could be more likely to develop symptoms under conditions of low social cohesion. This hypothesis might be tested by conducting surveys specifically examining the prevalence of BPD under different social conditions.

We do not know whether BPD has a differential prevalence between urban and rural settings. While research in the UK (Paykel et al., 2000) and in the USA (Robins & Regier, 1991) has found differences in the prevalence of mental disorders in general between urban and rural areas, such findings do not necessarily show that urban life is more stressful. However, a rural residence has been associated with a more likely recovery from mental illness, both in terms of decreasing symptomatology and improved life skills (Tirupati et al., 2010). We do not know whether these observations would apply to BPD.

Pinto et al. (2000) suggested that the absence of case reports or prevalence estimates of BPD in India prior to the late 1990s might suggest that the "close-knit" Indian culture has been protective against BPD. These authors thought that if they had examined patients in a rural rather than an urban setting, they would have found fewer cases than in their study, conducted in Mumbai. However, it is possible that such cases might not have been recognized. At this point, almost all research on the clinical prevalence of BPD in less developed countries comes from academic centers located in cities.

Another mechanism that could help account for differential prevalence of BPD is differences in the accumulation of *social capital*. This construct, introduced to sociology a century ago by Hanifan (1916, p. 132) was defined as "that in life which tends to make these tangible substances count for most in the daily lives of people, namely, goodwill, fellowship, mutual sympathy and social intercourse among a group of individuals and families." Social capital may be higher in rural communities than in urban environments, since members of smaller populations are more likely to form significant relationships with the people they know and see each day.

Social cohesion and social capital, associated with support from nuclear and extended family ties, are known to be generally protective against mental disorder (Gone & Kirmayer, 2010). Along the same lines, Giordano and Lindström (2011) have argued that "generalized trust", trust in the people and community around oneself, is the element of social capital that is most important for determining mental health outcomes, and that this sense of trust is fostered much more in a rural setting. These factors could help explain why BPD could be more prone to develop in less traditional settings, and why recovery from the disorder can sometimes be problematic. For the most chronic patients, who have lost all their social capital, the mental health system can become the only social network they can trust. However, more research is needed to substantiate this relationship.

Thus BPD is socially sensitive, occurs in specific social contexts, and is more likely to develop when social cohesion and social capital are compromised. These patients, who show unusual levels of susceptibility to their environment (Rioux et al., 2018), might therefore be considered, at least partly, as casualties of modernity and the rise of individualistic values. They are relatively unable to develop identities of their own in a society that fails to provide them with role models or adequate support.

Understanding the historical and cultural context of a disorder may be helpful in developing treatment plans. Borderline personality disorder patients have been shown to benefit from psychotherapy (Paris, 2020), but may also need sociotherapy (Tyrer, 2008). Clinicians who treat these cases should help patients to develop wider social networks, to build social capital, and to find social roles.

The Problem of Narcissism

Narcissistic Traits and Narcissistic Personality Disorder

Narcissistic personality disorder (NPD) is a controversial diagnosis. It came close to being eliminated from DSM-5 (*Diagnostic and Statistical Manual of Mental Disorders*), and is not listed in ICD-11 (*International Classification of Diseases*). The threat to drop NPD created dismay among several researchers (Miller & Campbell, 2010; Miller et al., 2010b) and expert clinicians (Pies, 2011; Ronningstam, 2011). Even *The New York Times* (Zanor, 2010) weighed in, suggesting wryly that narcissists don't like being ignored. Then, in June 2011, the DSM-5 work group reversed itself. This decision seems to have occurred because of feedback from influential clinicians that NPD is a useful construct that describes a characteristic group of patients seen in practice.

Yet research has found that NPD is common in the community and the clinic. The National Epidemiologic Survey on Alcohol and Related Conditions (NESARC) study reported a community prevalence of 6.2% (Stinson et al., 2008), but the revised estimate by Trull et al. (2010) reduced this rate to 1%, i.e., in about the same range as borderline personality disorder (BPD). A systematic review of several other published studies (Dhawan et al., 2010) also found a mean community prevalence of 1%. This number still makes NPD a highly prevalent disorder.

Given the fact that narcissism reduces help-seeking behaviors, one would expect a discrepancy between frequency in the community and in the clinic. In a large outpatient sample, one study reported a prevalence of 2.3% (Zimmerman et al., 2005). Also, clinical samples have a majority of females, while NPD may be more common in men (almost twice as frequent [Trull et al., 2010]). Perhaps the lower level of help-seeking in men can explain why some clinicians consider NPD to be relatively rare.

A large body of research has measured narcissistic traits in community populations (Campbell & Miller, 2011; Hermann et al., 2018; Levy et al., 2011). To measure the traits underlying a diagnosable disorder, the Narcissistic Personality Inventory (NPI), a measure particularly sensitive to grandiosity, has been widely used in research (Raskin & Terry, 1988). There is also a separate scale for pathological narcissism (Pincus et al., 2009). If NPD is essentially an amplified version of its underlying traits, this literature has clinical relevance. In fact, the findings show high levels of this trait that can be considered more or less equivalent to a diagnosis.

There has been some controversy about the validity of the NPI (Ackerman et al., 2011; Rosenthal et al., 2011; Trull, 2014). Specifically, the question is whether it actually measures self-esteem (Rosenthal & Hooley, 2010). Pathological narcissism differs from normal self-esteem: it is based on feelings of entitlement, with a failure to ground assessment of the self in objective accomplishments (Ronningstam, 2009).

Narcissistic personality disorder patients tend to make others suffer, but they also suffer as a consequence of their lack of understanding of other people. Narcissists can be fragile under stress. In fact, research shows many people with these traits are unhappy, lonely, and have poor social functioning (Miller et al., 2007). These outcomes could be a result of unsuccessful attempts to get others to meet their needs. Narcissistic personality disorder patients are more likely to be divorced and/or become unemployed, often leading to depressive symptoms (Ronningstam, 2011). In addition, while narcissism gradually declines with age (Foster et al., 2003), long-term interpersonal problems have cumulative effects that do not always go away with time. These are people who regularly lose jobs and romantic partners. While one recent study (that attracted attention in the media) suggested that subclinical narcissism protects people against depression (Papageorgiou et al., 2019), this need not be the case for those with pathological narcissism.

For clinical diagnosis, DSM-5, Section II, defines NPD in terms of meeting five out of nine criteria, which describe grandiosity, entitlement, and a lack of empathy. Due to a perceived lack of empirical support, ICD has never included this diagnosis in its manual. To diagnose NPD in DSM-5, Section III, the common features of all PDs (significant impairments in self and interpersonal functioning) must be present, manifest in self-functioning (excessive need for approval, grandiosity, entitlement) and interpersonal functioning (poor empathy and problematic intimacy). The associated trait domain for NPD is antagonism, associated with grandiosity (feelings of entitlement, either overt or covert, and self-centeredness, a belief that one is better than others) as well as attention-seeking (excessive seeking for admiration). These procedures follow the ideas of the DSM-5 work group that developed the Alternate Model of Personality Disorders (AMPD; Krueger et al., 2011). Their view was that since empirical data supports continuity between traits and disorders, the system can allow overall diagnosis of PDs, but use dimensional descriptors to account for individual variations in trait profiles.

The egosyntonic nature of narcissism, in which most problems in life are blamed on others, raises the question as to whether it can be measured accurately by self-report (Trull, 2014). Nonetheless, research on narcissism in the community has shown that these traits are continuous with the disorder, and can be measured reliably (Cain et al., 2008; Campbell & Miller, 2011). By and large, NPD is better supported by research than categories such as avoidant or obsessive compulsive PDs that were retained in the AMPD. Moreover, NPD is a clinically relevant construct (Paris, 2014).

In small doses, narcissistic traits can be adaptive and associated with ambition (Beck & Freeman, 2015). However, the more grandiose one is, the more likely that life will be disappointing. The Pathological Narcissism Inventory (PNI), which has a close relationship to the clinical diagnosis of NPD (Pincus et al., 2009), describes these dysfunctional levels (Miller & Campbell, 2010; Miller et al., 2009, 2010a; Miller & Maples, 2011). This gives us a rationale for applying research on narcissistic traits, both in clinical and community populations, to the study of diagnosable PDs (Cain et al., 2008).

There has been a controversy about the precise meaning of the narcissism construct, and whether it can be subdivided (Pincus & Lukowitsky, 2010). The claim is that NPD can take either a grandiose or a "covert-vulnerable" form (Cain et al., 2008; Miller et al., 2008). However, this idea runs the danger of unduly expanding the definition to include people who have grandiose fantasies rather than grandiose behaviors. The disorder lies on a continuum, but it is a stretch to use it to describe introverts who fantasize.

Although we lack prospective data on NPD, it is possible that some are more narcissistic when young, but mature enough to work their way past these traits. Nevertheless, if viewing oneself as superior to other people is not seen as a problem, it is harder to change (Ronningstam, 2009, 2011). Moreover, since NPD by itself is not necessarily associated with prominent symptoms, those who are affected may not seek treatment (Pincus & Lukowitsky, 2010).

Etiology

Behavioral genetic studies of NPD (Torgersen et al., 2000) and of narcissistic traits (Vernon et al., 2008) show that both have a heritable component, accounting for about 40% of the total variance. This suggests that people are not likely to develop NPD without first having a trait profile that makes them vulnerable to the disorder.

These findings also leave a large scope for environmental influence. Studies consistently show that the environmental component in personality and personality disorder is unshared, i.e., that siblings growing up in the same family do not necessarily have similar traits (Livesley et al., 1998). Moreover, if narcissistic traits precede NPD, these characteristics should be observable in childhood. This has been shown to be the case by several research groups (Hill & Roberts, 2011; Kerig & Stellwagen, 2010; Tackett & Mackrell, 2011; Thomaes et al., 2008).

Some of the specific psychological risk factors that amplify narcissistic traits to pathological levels suggest a role for permissiveness for grandiose narcissism, and for cold over-control in vulnerable narcissism (Horton, 2011; Horton et al., 2006). The first mechanism would be relevant to cultural trends that support parental and social reinforcement of grandiosity (Twenge & Campbell, 2009). These pathways raise the possibility of cohort effects on narcissism, mediated by sociocultural forces. In other words, we may be living in a culture that promotes narcissistic traits, at least in those who already have that profile.

Is Narcissism Increasing?

The social factors in narcissism have long been a topic of interest to historians (Lasch, 1979). In an individualistic society people are encouraged to admire themselves, often without any real accomplishments. Twenge (2011) has argued that, on the basis of cohort effects on NPI scores over time, narcissistic traits in the USA are increasing. If so, the prevalence of diagnosable NPD could also be increasing. While the increase is not large (effect size = 0.15), larger effects are rare in psychopathological research, probably because risk factors mainly affect a predisposed minority.

In surveys of university students, Twenge and Campbell (2009) compared data at different historical periods (30 years ago versus the present) and reported that contemporary subjects had higher NPI scores. Support for a cohort effect has also come from a meta-analysis of published studies, which found self-reported empathy among university students to be decreasing over several decades (Konrath, 2011).

These conclusions stimulated controversy. One obvious limitation is that published findings are generally based on self-reports of college-educated youth. The generalizability of findings from that population is always problematic, and observations in broader community samples are needed. Moreover, some researchers have failed to replicate the findings (Donnellan et al., 2009; Trzesniewski et al., 2008a, 2008b). These discrepancies probably reflect the use of different samples, with children from immigrant families being less likely to be narcissistic (Twenge, 2011).

However, Twenge (2011) found additional support for her hypothesis from other kinds of data. One involved the study of changes in cultural products. Thus, narcissistic themes have been increasing in the linguistic content of popular song lyrics, particularly after 2000 (DeWall et al., 2011). Obviously, these measures are indirect. More research in community populations is needed: narcissistic traits also need to be studied in populations at different socioeconomic levels and with different cultural backgrounds.

Twenge (2013) also argues that social media are in part responsible for increases in narcissism. She states that contrary to their original purpose (bringing people together), social media lead to disconnection and isolation in a world where direct personal communication is less valued. In a survey of adolescents, Twenge and Campbell (2018) stated that recent decreases in psychological well-being in this population tend to be associated with excessive use of smartphones. Twenge's group drew on data from a large-scale survey of American adolescents to support this conclusion (Twenge et al., 2019). They reported (p. 185) that "Cultural trends contributing to an increase in mood disorders and suicidal thoughts and behaviors since the mid-2000s, including the rise of electronic communication and digital media and declines in sleep duration, may have had a larger impact on younger people, creating a cohort effect." Again effect sizes are not large, and one would not expect that smartphones interfere with development in most adolescents, but have more effect on those who are already vulnerable.

Twenge's hypothesis of increasing cultural narcissism has a reasonable level of support from empirical evidence, and is consistent with a number of observations by social scientists and historians. Nevertheless, the strength of any cohort effect requires further research. In addition, even if these findings are replicated, we would still need to know whether they reflect a recent and dramatic change, or a gradual evolution over a longer period.

Twenge (2011) suggests a specific mechanism for a cohort effect, proposing that sociocultural changes in parenting practices influence levels of narcissism. Thus the mechanism behind an increase could depend on permissiveness, overindulgence, and the promotion of self-esteem independent of accomplishment. These problems would go beyond specific families, and derive from the culture at large. Twenge criticizes cultural trends in which people are encouraged to develop higher self-esteem without being expected to *do* things that make them deserving of praise. Twenge also notes that some day cares begin the day with a song in which children are asked to tell their caregivers how special they are. If everyone is special, though, no one is.

Narcissistic traits may also be more prevalent in modern societies than in traditional societies. Durvasula et al. (2001) developed a "Vanity Scale", which they administered to samples in the USA, New Zealand, India, and China. They found that subjects in India and China were less concerned about their physical appearance or their achievements than those living in the USA or New Zealand. NPI scores are higher in the USA than in Asia or the Middle East (Foster et al., 2003). Moreover, one study found that people who live in these countries share common perceptions of differences in national character that tend to support what have sometimes been considered stereotypes (Campbell et al., 2010). However, as globalization proceeds, these cross-cultural differences could be attenuated.

Modernity and Narcissism

Modernity has been the subject of intensive study by sociologists over several decades. The cultural changes and shifts in values associated with industrial and postindustrial society, associated with a decline in tradition and social norms, have been vast. These trends were already identified during the 19th and early 20th centuries, and may date back to the 18th-century Enlightenment (Giddens, 1991). It has long been hypothesized by social scientists that the characteristics of modern society promote a greater focus on self, as opposed to the collective (Markus & Kitayama, 1991).

Modernity could amplify narcissism by supporting the value of "expressive individualism" (Bellah et al., 1985). As traditional social structures weaken, people focus less on conforming to external expectations, and more on inner feelings. These changes have been accelerated by social and geographic mobility; as traditional social structures weaken, roots in family and community become more fragile. Moreover, as the social fabric weakens, the community provides less of a buffer against the vicissitudes of family life (Millon, 1993). Thus, as society modernizes, collective values become less important, and individual needs become more prominent, while basic human needs for connection and meaning are less easily met (Markus & Kitayama, 1994).

Individualism is the key aspect of modernity for psychological theory. The historical roots of individualism lie in the Enlightenment, but the term was first used in the early 19th century (Tocqueville, 1835/2000), gradually becoming a central value in contemporary society (Fischer, 2010). While autonomy and freedom yield many social and personal benefits (Deci & Ryan, 2002), individualism can carry a price. When the ultimate standard is what is good for oneself, rather than for family and/or community, people assess their actions on the basis of personal satisfaction, rather than by commitment to larger ideals (Rieff, 1966). This raises the question as to whether individualistic values, if held too strongly, inevitably shade into narcissism.

While modernity has its challenges, it is also associated with numerous positive benefits, from better physical health and decreased violence (Pinker, 2011) to increased well-being (Deci & Ryan, 2002). However, social change is a selection pressure that could have different effects on different people, with unique effects on vulnerable individuals (Rutter & Smith, 1995). Thus resilience to adverse life events is common, but is associated with characteristics that include an optimistic attitude, an ability to assess risks and consequences, and an ability to regulate emotions (Westphal & Bonnano, 2007). These characteristics could make people resilient, and be better equipped to deal with modernity and rapid social change. In contrast, individuals with personality traits that do not promote resilience would be at greater risk for developing mental disorders (Rutter & Smith, 1995). Thus modernity could be more positive for individuals with characteristics that help them to cope with change, but negative for those whose vulnerability makes coping more difficult.

Patients with PDs have many problematic traits, and can be described in the Five Factor Model as having low agreeableness, low conscientiousness, and high neuroticism (Costa & Widiger, 2013). These traits, which are associated with narcissism (Miller et al., 2010a), may interfere with adaptive responses to social stressors. In NPD, grandiosity can make people vulnerable to adversity, since behind a mask of arrogance, pathological narcissism fails to address inner emotional needs, which, when frustrated, present as rage and/or withdrawal (Ronningstam, 2011). This raises a question concerning the extent to which NPD patients require social structures and networks.

There is a universal human need for attachment, in both interpersonal and social contexts (Baumeister & Leary, 1995). This observation is consistent with sociological concepts, which since the time of Durkheim (1897/1997) have linked psychological distress to social alienation and loss of social cohesion. The concept of "social capital" (Putnam, 2000) is a more recent formulation of the positive influence of social networks on psychological functioning. However, when social capital is insufficient, people may turn to themselves for affirmation. This can lead to a scenario in which poor social supports reinforce narcissism.

These pathways are not specific to NPD. Similar mechanisms have been invoked to explain increases in the prevalence of other personality disorders. In addition, NPD can likely develop only in people with specific temperamental profiles.

Since narcissism is associated with individualist values, it should be most prevalent in societies, and in subgroups within a society, that have most strongly embraced that worldview. Twenge's (2011) review of empirical studies argues for a cohort effect dating from the 1980s. However, the cultural changes affecting narcissistic traits go back much further.

Narcissism is hardly a new historical phenomenon. No purely collectivist traditional society has ever been described; in every historical period, ambitious people have indulged in self-display and sought fame and attention (Baudry, 1986). What is unique about modern societies is that they promote values that encourage narcissism in everyone, not just in an elite (Lasch, 1979). Even if these trends have accelerated in recent decades, most observers of modernity (e.g., Giddens, 1991) have suggested a turning point around the year 1900.

If the effects of modernity were gradual and cumulative, they may not have been easily observed until they reached a tipping point. Increased interest in narcissism among psychotherapists and social critics dates from the 1960s and 1970s, and these observations could be related to the social changes that characterized those decades (Marwick, 2000). Some of the most important clinical theories about NPD, including the work of psychoanalysts such as Kohut (1970) and Kernberg (1976) also date from this era.

The historian Christopher Lasch introduced the term "cultural narcissism" to describe how excessively individualistic values affect contemporary society. Lasch (1979) hypothesized that modern society encourages individuals to focus on self and to loosen ties to community, and that contemporary culture has come to focus on fame, celebrity, and riches (as opposed to duty, honor, and service). Lasch further suggested that social developments in the course of the 20th century amplified narcissistic traits, producing fragile self-concepts, fear of commitments and lasting relationships, a dread of aging, and an excessive admiration for celebrity.

Others, including popular journalists (Wolfe, 1976), have described similar social trends. The political philosopher Amitzai Etzioni (1993) saw modern society as atomizing the individual and ignoring the universal human need for social networks and connections. Putnam (2000) saw modernity as reducing *social capital*, i.e., a loss of meaningful connections, making people turn to self rather than to community. Low social capital may also increase the risk for divorce, since too much is expected of one intimate relationship. All these processes describe an individualism that became extreme, shading into narcissism, and leading to social disconnection.

Narcissism and Psychotherapy

To understand the relation between narcissism and psychotherapy, we need to consider the social role of psychological treatment (Cushman, 1990). Talking therapy did not exist prior to a little over 100 years ago. That was the same time as the acceleration of modernity – which may not be a coincidence. The rise of psychotherapy may have been in part an attempt to deal with problems created by modernity, specifically a less predictable social environment (Gellner, 1993).

Psychological treatment is a product of modern culture that has, in turn, had a profound effect on contemporary values. Over 50 years ago, the sociologist Phillip Rieff (1966) described the development of a "therapy culture" linked to radical individualism. Rieff noted that social virtue had become less of an ideal in modern culture, and that the well-being of the individual had become paramount over that of society as a whole. He also observed that a "therapeutic" orientation makes all truths contingent and negotiable, undermining shared social values.

Other commentators have reached similar conclusions. The psychologist Phillip Cushman (1990) argued that modernity produces an "empty self", shorn of social meaning, and strongly criticized psychotherapy for promoting individualistic values over social connections. The sociologist Frank Furedi (2004) elaborated on these ideas in a book critiquing the development of a "therapeutic culture", in which self-esteem becomes more important than social commitment.

Most commentators on "therapeutic culture" have been critics of psychoanalytic therapies, which have a tendency to encourage self-absorption (Gellner, 1993). However, not all forms of psychotherapy are the same. This problem could be less true for cognitive behavioral therapy (Beck & Freeman, 2015) and interpersonal therapy (Klerman & Weissman, 1993), whose theories and methods are oriented to the current social environment.

Nonetheless, the inner dynamic of all psychotherapies encourages patients to look inside the self as a way of dealing with the outside world (Furedi, 2004). For those who are overly concerned with social demands, focus on the self might lead to a better balance. However, for those who are already grandiose and seeking of attention, talking therapy could become as much part of the problem as a part of the solution. In this way classical elements of psychotherapy such as empathy and unconditional positive regard (Rogers, 1951) can be double-edged. Talking about oneself to a therapist who listens carefully and offers support might even be considered a narcissist's dream. In this way, some forms of psychological treatment risk supporting the very traits that lead to dysfunction.

We do not know whether existing psychotherapies are effective for the treatment of NPD. Several psychoanalysts have described approaches to the treatment of narcissism (Kernberg, 1987; Kohut, 1977; Ronningstam, 2009). There are five chapters on psychotherapy in the *Handbook of Narcissism and Narcissistic Personality Disorder* (Campbell & Miller, 2011) that include transference-focused psychotherapy, attachment therapy, schema therapy, cognitive behavioral therapy, and dialectical behavior therapy. However, none of these chapters are evidence-based: none of the methods has ever been tested in clinical trials or shown to be effective in samples of NPD patients.

It is true that treatment research for most PDs (with the exception of the borderline category) is generally thin. Nevertheless, the reputation of patients with NPD for being difficult may not be unwarranted. There is some evidence that narcissism interferes with psychotherapy (Ogrodniczuk et al., 2009). However, we need more empirical research on this patient population, particularly concerning the effect of narcissism on psychotherapy process and outcome.

The difficulties associated with the psychological treatment of NPD could relate to the general factors that research shows to impede good outcome, such as a poor therapeutic alliance and a tendency to externalize problems (Orlinsky et al., 1994). It is also possible that psychotherapy, if it focuses exclusively on the interests of individuals, carries an *intrinsic* danger of reinforcing narcissism (Paris, 2013). While no empirical studies have directly examined how therapists use the concept of self-esteem, models that increase regard for the self, although more characteristic of popular psychology than of evidence-based practice, have had an influence on the thinking of many clinicians (Furedi, 2004; Satel & Sommers, 2005).

Treatment for patients with narcissistic traits and/or NPD may require unique methods that have yet to be developed. Generic therapies developed for common mental disorders are not consistently useful for PDs, as has been shown to be the case for BPD, which does not respond well to "treatment as usual" (Paris, 2010a). Rather, BPD has been found to remit with highly structured therapies that are specifically designed to deal with emotion dysregulation and impulsivity, such as dialectical behavior therapy (Linehan, 1993). Identification of traits that could be targeted might also help to define the elements that need to be included in a specific therapy for NPD. Thus treatment might need to offer ways to challenge grandiosity effectively, and to provide tools to reduce vulnerability. Patients with NPD may also need a better balance between individual goals and social attachments. Development of a model based on these principles could then be followed by clinical trials to determine efficacy.

Suggestions for Further Research

The proposal that increasing cultural narcissism is promoting the development of NPD and associated traits has some support from empirical data, and from the social science literature, but requires much more research. Thus, measures such as NPI scores need to be examined more systematically, and move beyond convenience samples to large community populations, cross-cultural samples, and prospective research in population cohorts.

Second, the hypothesis that therapy runs the risk of promoting narcissism has also not been examined empirically. While narcissism probably makes psychotherapy more difficult, studies are needed to examine the effects of therapy on these traits, particularly in extended courses of treatment and in different modalities. The use of standard measures of narcissism in psychotherapy research could shed light on these questions. Studies of how therapists of different persuasions view the problem of self-esteem might also be illuminating. Finally, the suggestion for a new method of psychotherapy specifically designed to modify narcissism could be the basis of a long-term research project.

These lines of investigation would all take time. While awaiting more definitive data, therapists and theoreticians need to place the problem of narcissism in a historical and sociocultural perspective that goes beyond individual life narratives. Psychotherapists cannot change the culture and society in which we live, but they can be aware of its contradictions, and avoid promoting values that have the potential to support narcissism.

Chapter

7

Antisocial Personality Disorder

Definition and Diagnosis

Antisocial personality disorder (ASPD) has been an accepted category of mental illness, albeit with different names, for two centuries. Antisocial personality disorder is a highly egosyntonic disorder that fits well within a PD construct. The idea that there is a form of mental disorder characterized by callousness and criminality is fairly universal across cultures. In psychiatry many different terms: "moral insanity", "psychopathy", or "sociopathy" have been used to describe this pattern (Berrios, 1993). The term psychopathy is still frequently used to describe a more severe form of the disorder.

The definition of ASPD in the *Diagnostic and Statistical Manual of Mental Disorders* (DSM-5), Section II requires a pervasive pattern of disregard and violation of the rights of others, as indicated by at least three of the following: criminal actions, deceitfulness, impulsivity, aggressiveness, recklessness, irresponsibility, and lack of remorse. This pattern must have begun before age 15. In DSM-5, Section III, the category is built up from profiles that reflect the same groups of traits. In the *International Classification of Diseases* (ICD-11), the diagnosis as such does not appear, but patients can be described as high on traits of dissociality and disinhibition.

Since its third edition, the DSM system has required that ASPD be preceded by a prior diagnosis of conduct disorder. This rule is based on research first published decades ago by Robins (1966). However, while the symptoms of conduct disorder are essentially early versions of the phenomena seen in adult ASPD, only one-third of cases of conduct disorder go on to develop ASPD (Zoccolillo et al., 1992). Therefore the diagnosis of ASPD in DSM-5 cannot be made until the patient is at least 18 years of age. (This rule has led to confusion among clinicians, some of whom think that it applies to all PDs, which it does not.)

Antisocial behavior in children has a different outcome depending on age of onset (Moffitt et al., 2001). Those with an early onset and callous unemotional traits (a marker for psychopathy) are most likely to develop ASPD in adulthood. In contrast, those with an adolescent onset and an absence of callous unemotional traits have a much better prognosis, and do not usually develop adult ASPD. In twin samples (Button et al., 2005), the first group had symptoms that were more heritable, while the second group showed more influence of shared environment.

In order to diagnose ASPD in adults, consistent criminal behavior is a crucial feature. It is therefore not surprising that from two-thirds to three-quarters of male prison populations meet criteria (De Brito & Hodgins, 2009). Since delinquency and criminality are behaviors that can more readily be measured, they have been used as markers for ASPD in epidemiological research.

The construct of "psychopathy" places more emphasis on personality characteristics that may accompany criminality, particularly manipulativeness and interpersonal exploitativeness (Cleckley, 1976). Coid and Ulrich (2010) suggest that psychopathy is a more severe form of ASPD. In DSM-5, this subgroup is described as having a specifier: *callous unemotional traits*, a feature that can also be observed in many conduct disordered children (Kerig & Stellwagen, 2010).

A group of researchers led by the Canadian psychologist Robert Hare have argued that there are two factors in psychopathy, one describing chronic criminality and the other pathological interpersonal behavior, and criticized the definition of ASPD for describing only the first of these (Hart & Hare, 1996). They also noted that when both dimensions are considered, only a minority of criminals meet diagnostic criteria for psychopathy.

This construct has been popular in forensic work, especially given the wide use of Hare's Psychopathy Checklist, revised (PCL-R), an interview measure that guides clinicians and investigators to make the diagnosis (Hare, 2003). Thus a large proportion of published research is on the construct of psychopathy rather than on ASPD.

Prevalence

Clear-cut behavioral criteria have made it practical to examine ASPD in research, and it was the only PD included in the Epidemiological Catchment Area (ECA) study (Robins & Regier, 1991), as well as in the National Comorbidity Study Replication (NCS-R; Kessler et al., 2005), both of which determined the prevalence of psychiatric disorders in a number of sites in the USA.

The prevalence of ASPD is similar in several English-speaking countries: in two American studies, the ECA study and the NCS-R it was, respectively, 2.4% and 3.5%. In a Canadian study (Bland et al., 1998), it was 3.7%; in a New Zealand study (Oakley-Browne et al., 1989), it was 3.1%. In Trull et al.'s (2010) revised estimates based on data from the National Epidemiologic Survey on Alcohol and Related Conditions (NESARC), its prevalence was 3.7%. Thus ASPD is a common disorder in the community, even if nonforensic psychiatrists see it only rarely. The reason is that its pathology is egosyntonic, and many consultations are initiated by lawyers rather than by patients.

Antisocial personality disorder is correlated with demographic variables, and is more common in youth, in males, and in lower socioeconomic classes (Black, 2008). The association with male gender is very consistent, the disorder being five to seven times more common in men than women. The association with lower socioeconomic status is also consistent, as is a strong negative relationship to education. The symptoms of ASPD tend to "burn out" over time, confirming its strong association with youth. However, many patients continue to have serious problems holding onto jobs or relationships (Black, 2015).

Antisocial personality disorder does not show differential prevalence by race; nor have researchers found differences between ethnic groups living in the same city (Black, 2008). The ECA study reported an increased prevalence in urban as opposed to rural sites, and one city (St. Louis) had a particularly high rate (Robins & Regier, 1991). The NCS-R did not find urban-rural differences, but ASPD showed regional differences (Kessler et al., 2005) that could be due to the migration of antisocial individuals, or to effects of social risk factors.

Antisocial personality disorder can be found in all societies, but its prevalence shows important cross-cultural differences that provide strong evidence for the role of social factors. The most important data comes from samples from urban and rural areas of Taiwan (Compton et al., 1991; Hwu et al., 1989), which had unusually low prevalence of ASPD, ranging from 0.03% to 0.14%. There is evidence that these low rates also apply to mainland China (Tseng, 2001), to India (Gupta & Mattoo, 2012), to Japan (Sato & Takeichi, 1993), and to several countries in Africa (Rossier et al., 2008).

The second important line of epidemiological evidence pointing to social factors in ASPD is that it increased in prevalence in Western countries after World War II (Rutter & Smith, 1995). Both the ECA and NCS-R studies estimated that the lifetime prevalence of ASPD in the United States nearly doubled among young people in 15 years. Rapid increases in prevalence of mental disorders over short periods of time can, with few exceptions, only be accounted for by changes in the social environment.

Etiology

There is consistent evidence that biological risk factors are implicated in ASPD: behavior genetic studies in twin samples confirm a heritability close to 50% (Werner et al., 2015). Adoption studies also show that criminality in a biological parent is a risk factor for criminality in a child (Crowe, 1974; Mednick et al., 1984). Biological markers, i.e., loss of neuronal areas that are visible on fRMI, are also associated with criminality (Raine, 2013). However, these findings may apply more consistently to severe cases with psychopathy.

Some of the most consistent biological findings are neuropsychological (Sutker et al., 1993). Antisocial individuals fail to develop conditioned responses to stimuli related to fear (Dolan & Park, 2002). These observations concord with clinical reports that antisocial patients have a lack of normal fearfulness, and an inability to learn from negative experiences (Cleckley, 1976). Decades ago, Eysenck and Gudjonsson (1989) suggested that reduced capacity for conditioning is a diathesis for antisocial behavior. There are conditions under which fearlessness can be adaptive, and antisocial individuals in the military may function well in combat, but not in peacetime.

Kagan (1994) labeled the constitutional factor in antisocial personality as "uninhibited temperament", in contrast to the behavioral inhibition seen in those with anxious traits. Farrington (1993) also concluded that an inhibited temperament is a protective factor against criminality. Disinhibition would not be sufficient by itself to cause criminality, but could be a necessary precondition for its development.

Studies of the personality dimensions of antisocial patients have demonstrated low neuroticism, low agreeableness, and low conscientiousness in the Five Factor Model (Costa & Widiger, 2013). Since these dimensions of personality have a genetic component, they indirectly reflect some of the temperamental factors behind ASPD.

Other biological factors might be associated with comorbidities. One of the most prominent is alcoholism and substance use (Werner et al., 2015). Another is attention deficit hyperactive disorder (ADHD) – long-term follow-ups of hyperactive children show that about a third of these cases develop significant antisocial behavior in adulthood (Hechtman, 2016).

The strong gender difference in the prevalence of ASPD also implicates biological factors. If there is one finding in psychology you can count on, it is that criminality is much more common in men (Moffitt et al., 2001). The higher rate could be due in part to greater physical aggression, which is, as shown almost half a century ago, the most consistent gender difference between male and female children (Maccoby & Jacklin, 1974). Moreover, similarly high proportions of men are seen in ADHD and substance use.

The large-scale prospective study carried out in St. Louis, Missouri, by Lee Robins (1966) tested the hypothesis that specific symptoms in childhood are the precursors of ASPD. Over 500 children seen at a child guidance clinic were followed as adults. One of the principal findings was that only those children whose delinquency had begun prior to adolescence could be diagnosed later as "sociopathic". This observation was later confirmed in a British study (West & Farrington, 1973).

We do not understand why some children with conduct disorder go on to develop ASPD, while others do not. Even if we cannot predict outcome precisely, there are statistical associations. Robins (1966) found that in two-thirds of the families of children who later developed sociopathy, both parents

had psychiatric or behavioral problems. The most frequent and most important was antisocial behavior in the father. (There was also a higher frequency of
antisocial behavior in the mother, as well as more parental alcoholism.)

These findings may reflect genetic factors common to antisocial parents
and their antisocial offspring. However, having an antisocial parent is also an
environmental risk for children. One should not be surprised, for example, to
find that severe family dysfunction is associated with being raised by an
antisocial parent. Traumatic experiences might be more common in children
growing up in such families. Pollack et al. (1990) found that, in conjunction
with parental alcoholism, physical abuse was the strongest antecedent of adult
antisocial behavior. Also, family dysfunction does not necessarily end when
fathers leave, since the women who pick these partners have psychopathology
of their own.

Robins (1966) also noted that the family structure of children who
developed ASPD leads to a failure of parents to discipline and supervise their
children, a finding confirmed in a British study (West & Farrington, 1973).
Parental discord made no independent contribution to the risk when pathology in the father was taken into account. However, separation or loss of a
parent was an independent risk factor. Only one-third of ASPD cases were
raised by two parents, an unusual rate at the time when the children were
originally assessed (90 years ago). There was also a positive relationship
between sociopathy and large family size.

Other studies examining risks for delinquency and crime present a similar
picture. For example, in a prospective study in the Boston area (McCord,
1978), the most powerful predictor of delinquency was parental instability,
while the presence of a relationship to a stable and affectionate parent was a
strong protective factor. In the British prospective study (West & Farrington,
1973), the risk factors were low family income, large family size, parental
criminality, low intelligence, and lack of discipline and control from parents.

All these findings point to family dysfunction as the most important
psychological risk factor for ASPD. The most likely mechanism by which
dysfunctional families promote psychopathy is through a decreased frequency
or inconsistency of punishment, with an absence of clear consequences and
limits for children's behavior.

However, cross-cultural differences in prevalence, as well as the recent
increase in the prevalence of ASPD in North America, point to a crucial role
for social pathology in this disorder. Social structures affect prevalence by
lowering or raising the threshold at which other risks influence the development of disorders. East Asian cultures with low prevalence must be protective
against ASPD, probably through interfaces between culture and family structure. Such families have characteristics that present a veritable mirror image of
the risk factors: fathers are strong and authoritative, expectations of children
are high, and family loyalty is prized. In the Robins study, there was a

particularly low rate of ASPD in Jewish subjects, which she attributed to their strong family structures. Of course, highly traditional families have their own difficulties, and their repressive style could make children susceptible to other forms of personality disorder.

Contrary to popular opinion, poverty does not explain the prevalence of antisocial behavior. Robins found no relationship between lower socioeconomic status and sociopathy, independent of criminality in the father. Poverty is not related to crime when families are functioning well. As Vaillant and Vaillant (1981) found in a long-term follow-up of an inner-city sample, most people raised in poverty work to make their lives better, and never turn to crime. This conclusion is supported by another finding from the Robins study, that membership in gangs was only a risk factor for children who already came from dysfunctional families.

The greatest increase in the prevalence of both criminality and ASPD in the West since World War II has taken place in the face of unprecedented prosperity (Rutter & Smith, 1995). It is more likely that family dysfunction, acting as a mediating factor for social influences, is most responsible for an increasing prevalence of ASPD.

The vulnerability to ASPD is probably more widely distributed than antisocial behavior itself. Underlying impulsive traits do not attain dysfunctional proportions if they are "contained" by a strong family and by social structures. Overt antisocial behavior will only emerge in the presence of family dysfunction and social disintegration.

Interactions between Predispositions and Familial Stressors

Biologically rooted temperamental variations, as well as family dysfunction, are necessary conditions for the development of ASPD, but that does not make them sufficient. Rather the disorder derives from interactions between temperament and psychosocial risks. The strongest data comes from longitudinal studies in which stressors can be accurately measured prior to the development of the full disorder (Jaffee et al., 2004; Moffitt, 2005). Some research has found that antisocial tendencies can be predicted in early childhood (Caspi et al., 1996; Kim-Cohen et al., 2003).

In the study by Robins (1966), having a father who has psychopathy, whether living with the family or not, was the strongest predictor of psychopathy in a child. However, if parents have similar behavioral disorders, transmission of traits to children could be largely genetic. We need a method to separate correlations between a stressful environment and the partially heritable traits underlying ASPD. Thus, research needs to examine these relationships in twin samples, allowing us to control for genetic risk.

Drawing on the Dunedin study (a longitudinal follow-up of a birth cohort in New Zealand), as well as the Environmental Risk (E-Risk) study in the UK, Wertz et al. (2018) reported that both genetic and environmental factors were a predictor of antisocial behavior. Behavior genetic studies use twin samples to determine the influence of heritability, shared environment, and unshared environment. Application of this procedure yields unique results (Jaffee, 2017). Unlike most other mental disorders, shared environmental variance plays a significant role in ASPD (Werner et al., 2015). Nevertheless, these nonheritable psychosocial factors come from families, from neighborhoods, and from society at large.

In twin studies that examine both heritable and nonheritable factors, about half the variance affecting antisocial behavior is driven by the shared environment. In a longitudinal study of 1,116 twin pairs in the UK, the E-Risk study, environmental factors had a large and separate contribution to the variance (Jaffee et al., 2003). The risks were primarily related to abusive parenting and highly dysfunctional families and increased when the father continued to live with the family. Finally, the mothers of antisocial children were often depressed, further increasing psychosocial risk.

It is nearly universal that children who develop conduct disorder and are diagnosed as adults with ASPD come from families with poor and inconsistent parenting (Jaffee, 2003, Moffitt et al., 2001). These families also tend to be *coercive* (Snyder, 2015), i.e., authoritarian and insensitive rather than understanding and supportive, and are often marked by maltreatment associated with both physical abuse and serious neglect (VanZomeren-Dohm et al., 2015).

In a large-scale longitudinal study of high-risk children raised in families marked by socioeconomic deprivation, Farrington (1993) documented how childhood antisocial behavior and a constellation of adversities, including poverty, large families, ineffective child rearing, antisocial parents, parental disharmony and separation predicted antisocial behaviors at age 18. The most frequent outcomes in adolescence were violence, dishonesty, heavy drinking, drug abuse, reckless driving, sexual promiscuity, and an unstable job record. When Farrington and Welsh (2008) extended the follow-up to age 30, they noted a persistence of antisocial behavior.

Even so, as pointed out in a systematic review by Moffitt (2005), until it can be shown that relationships are truly causal, research will be "stuck" at a stage of identifying risk factors rather than etiological pathways. To account for a complex developmental pathway, we need to apply a biopsychosocial model to ASPD. This means building a model that takes into account interfaces and interactions between heritable predispositions and environmental stressors.

However, the mechanisms through which genes and environment interact remain unclear. Moreover, while interactive gene-environmental approaches are crucial they are complicated. For example, antisocial children are much more likely to elicit negative reactions to their behavior from their families (Rutter & Rutter, 1993). Epigenetic methods might offer a pathway, but this approach to child development has not produced many consistent findings. Another method is to obtain polygenetic risk scores (summing the effects of many genes), but this line of research tends to identify many polymorphisms, each only having a small effect. It will probably take many decades to unravel these knots and develop a useful and predictive causal model.

Societal Factors in Antisocial Personality Disorder

Research has documented large differences in ASPD prevalence between different countries and different cultural settings. In most Western countries, the population prevalence is around 1%–3%. Yet cultures that actively discourage antisocial behavior, such as a traditional Confucian society, have the capacity to suppress ASPD.

Although ASPD increased in prevalence in Western societies after World War II, in the last two decades, in spite of further societal upheavals, the crime rate in developed countries has gone down (Farrell et al., 2014). The reason for this fall, accompanied by a reduction in child abuse and neglect (Finkelhor et al., 2005), is not known. Such changes cannot be genetically based, but could be due to either improved quality of parenting or a better social climate. A vast body of evidence shows that whatever problems are obvious in the short-term, over the long-term, human societies are becoming more fair to all their members, and poverty is much less severe than it once was (Pinker, 2011, 2018).

In building a model of social risk factors for ASPD, we need to consider the neighborhoods in which children are raised (Jennings & Fox, 2012). Some seem to encourage rather than discourage antisocial behavior. It has often been thought that people with limited opportunities are more likely to turn to crime. Yet most children of poverty do not embrace these options. There are protective factors here, including both family support (Schofield et al., 2012) and social capital (Bourdieu, 1986).

Another idea one sees in recent years is that social media can support antisocial behavior, and encourage people with traits in a "dark triad" of psychopathy, narcissism, and Machiavellianism to do things to hurt other people (Craker & March, 2016). However, evidence for this hypothesis is thin; since the invention of writing there have always been newer technologies that can be used as a means of expression for antisocial individuals. Thus society can encourage or discourage PDs, but it cannot produce them by itself,

Implications for Outcome and Treatment

Antisocial patients usually improve over time, and are less likely to show criminal behavior past middle age (Black, 2015). Longitudinal research on adult development in normal cohorts documents reductions in impulsivity over time (Vaillant, 1977). The explanation could be, in part, that continuous brain maturation during adulthood is associated with changes in levels of specific neurotransmitters. Improvements in neurochemical balances, particularly related to the serotonergic system, might decrease impulsivity. A second explanation of the "burnout" of ASPD could be that however slow they are to learn from experience, antisocial individuals can gradually undergo a degree of change.

Of any personality disorder, the treatment of ASPD offers the most pessimistic prospects for success. Attempts to treat antisocial patients have generally involved either individual and group psychotherapies, or creating artificial environments in the form of "therapeutic communities". However, there is no evidence that any of these methods has any lasting effects.

Although devoted clinicians in forensic settings continue to apply clinical skills to antisocial inmates, there have been no convincing clinical trials showing that any method of therapy is consistently effective for this population. This was so a few decades ago (Dolan & Coid, 1993) and remains so today. Antisocial individuals rarely ask to change their behavior. If anything, they usually demand that society change. This is the main reason why treatment prospects for this disorder remain bleak.

Other Personality Disorders

8

This chapter will consider PD categories for which research data is less abundant. It will not review research on the "Cluster A" disorders in the *Diagnostic and Statistical Manual of Mental Disorders* (DSM-5) (schizoid, paranoid, and schizotypal), since these conditions are best understood as subclinical variants of schizophrenia, and are classified in the Alternative Model of Personality Disorder (AMPD) as a single category (schizotypal PD).

The "Cluster C" PDs listed in DSM-5, Section II (avoidant, compulsive, and dependent) are loosely linked by traits associated with anxiety. When anxious traits interfere either with the capacity to work or the ability to develop intimate relationships, one should diagnose a PD. However, dependent PD was dropped in the AMPD system in Section III. This condition has been rarely researched; the main exception has been the work of Robert Bornstein (2005). Epidemiological studies suggest this category is rare in the community, at only 0.3% (Trull et al., 2010).

Obsessive compulsive personality disorder (OCPD) is retained in both sections of DSM-5. The *International Classification of Diseases* (ICD-11) describes it as rooted in a trait domain of "anankastia". Probably because OCPD lacks a clear separation from its underlying traits, the National Epidemiologic Survey on Alcohol and Related Conditions (NESARC) (Grant et al., 2004) reported an amazingly high prevalence of 7.9%. Once again, Trull et al. (2010) raised the bar, and reduced this estimate to a much more reasonable estimate of 1.9%. Behaviorial genetic studies of OCPD suggest it may not belong in an anxious cluster, and that its traits do not overlap with avoidance and dependence (Livesley et al., 1998).

Avoidant personality disorder (AVPD) is characterized by a hypersensitivity to rejection that leads to avoidance of relationships. Avoidant personality disorder was the most frequent diagnosis (14.7%) in the clinical sample studied by Zimmerman et al. (2005). Trull et al. (2010) found AVPD affects about 1% of the general population.

DSM-5, Section II requires the presence at least four of seven criteria for a diagnosis of AVPD: avoidance of interpersonal contacts at work;

unwillingness to get involved with people unless certain of being liked; restraint in intimate relationships; preoccupation with criticism and rejection; inhibition in new interpersonal situations; view of self as inept, unappealing, or inferior; reluctance to take risks or engage in new activities. In Section III, AVPD is defined in a similar way, but the diagnosis is built up from trait profiles (negative affectivity and detachment). Similar traits of negative affectivity are listed in ICD-11 and correspond to this definition.

Biological Risk Factors for Anxious Personality Disorders

The empirical literature on these disorders is thin (Weinbrecht et al., 2016). However, the diagnosis of AVPD is highly comorbid with symptomatic anxiety disorders, particularly social anxiety disorder (Lampe, 2016). Notably, AVPD strongly overlaps with generalized social anxiety; twin studies show common genetic effects (Stein et al., 2002; Welander-Vatn et al., 2019). Thus a common diathesis can lead either to anxious symptoms, anxious personality traits, or both. Most of these findings can be understood on the basis of inborn differences in the intensity of social anxiety.

In a classic series of studies, Kagan (1994) described a specific form of anxious temperament, which he labeled "behavioral inhibition". The operational definition of behavioral inhibition involves unusual levels of shyness in infancy, as demonstrated by anxiety and withdrawal when faced with unfamiliar social stimuli. Kagan found that this trait shows a strong genetic influence, with a heritability of about 50%. Behavioral inhibition is also associated with high levels of physiological arousal, associated with the broader domain of neuroticism.

Kagan studied cohorts of infants with behavioral inhibition, and then followed them up, first at age 7, and then at age 13. In three-quarters of the cases, they continued to have this trait. Unfortunately we do not know to what extent behavioral inhibition continues into adulthood.

Most children eventually manage to "grow out" of shyness. If there is a subgroup in which behavioral inhibition persists into adulthood, there could be two explanations. One is that high levels of traits are least likely to remit spontaneously. Another possibility is that anxious temperament can improve when parents expose their children to anxiety-provoking social situations. (Behavioral inhibition is more common in younger than in older siblings, which could reflect the tendency of parents to be more protective of younger children.) Kagan believes that children are more likely to overcome behavioral inhibition if their families encourage and help them to do so. About 25% of Kagan's cohort no longer showed behavioral inhibition at age seven.

Psychological Risk Factors for Anxious Personality Disorders

Compared with the large amount of research on borderline personality disorder (BPD), there have been few empirical studies on the psychological risk factors for disorders in the anxious cluster. However, like other PDs, anxious cluster disorders develop due to interactions between temperament and experience. If families do not encourage a shy child, either because of lack of interest, or because they share the child's fears, then these personality traits can become more stable and more dysfunctional.

In a retrospective study of patients with AVPD, Arbel and Stravynski (1991) described histories of an unsupportive family life, with few demonstrations of parental love and pride. These characteristics may resemble a style of parenting that Parker (1983) has termed "affectionless control". While perceptions of family environment can also reflect temperament, patients with AVPD may begin life with a biological diathesis, after which a lack of parental support amplifies an anxious temperament.

The psychosocial risks for AVPD might be accounted for by attachment theory (Bowlby, 1969), a model that aims to explain normal and abnormal bonding in children and adults. Its basic premise is that attachment between children and their caretakers is a biological program adapted for survival. "Anxious attachment" in children is characterized by an abnormal fear of separation. However, while Bowlby hypothesized that this phenomenon reflects problems in parenting, he failed to consider that variation in sensitivity to parental styles is a heritable trait. In a twin study, Crawford et al. (2007) showed that insecure attachment has a similar level of heritability to most PDs (40%).

Attachment theory has stimulated a large amount of empirical research (Cassidy & Shaver, 2018). In general, attachment styles can be classified into secure, anxious-preoccupied, dismissive-avoidant, and fearful-avoidant. The stability of these attachment patterns, as well as their relationship to child-rearing practices, are subjects of controversy. Some children with avoidant or anxious patterns are overprotective but others have normal parenting (Kagan, 1994).

While a "secure" style of attachment has been considered normative, it is not the only type associated with good functioning. Kagan (1989) criticized attachment theory for its culturally based assumption that "love" is the most important element of normal development and mental health. For example, an avoidant attachment style (in which the child shows little reaction to the absence or return of the mother) is associated with good functioning in Scandinavia, where the culture gives greater value to emotional control.

Social Risk Factors for Anxious Cluster Personality Disorders

An anxious temperament will be more adaptive in some social structures than in others. In "the environment of evolutionary adaptiveness", strong attachments to caretakers were essential to avoid predation (Bowlby, 1969). In addition, early human groups developed as small communities surrounded by hostile outsiders, so that the avoidance of strangers was necessary. Even in modern societies, there are many real dangers, for both children and adults, from contact with strangers.

The structures of traditional societies tend to promote these traits. Cohesive family and social structures found in traditional societies reward dependent traits, and punish excessive individualism. In these settings, individuals with avoidant and/or dependent traits more readily fit in to the expectations of the community, and will not be considered pathological.

For example, the Japanese are higher as a group on dimensions of introversion and neuroticism (Iwawaki et al., 1977), and are more likely to have social phobias (Kirmayer, 1991). We would therefore expect to find that they have more personality traits associated with social avoidance and dependence. This pattern might apply to any society with high social cohesion.

Problems arise when these traits are prominent in people growing up in modern societies that require individualism and autonomy. Successful individuals have to manage frequent interactions with strangers. Unless families help children with behavioral inhibition overcome their difficulties, they can become socially maladaptive, since as adults, they will not be able to find employment or a family on their own. Discordance between avoidant traits and social expectations can create a vicious cycle: the more the individual is unable to cope with social demands, the more these traits are amplified.

The social factors in anxious cluster personality disorders may not be qualitatively different from those in other categories. Social disintegration and rapid social change, by increasing requirements for individual autonomy, create demands that are most likely to make traits characterized by either impulsivity or avoidance maladaptive. In both cases, the absence of securely available social networks in modern cultures undermine some of the protective factors against psychopathology. However, in the absence of research data, we do not know whether there are cross-cultural differences or cohort effects on the prevalence of anxious PDs.

Unspecified Personality Disorder

The most common form of PD in clinical practice is personality disorder, unspecified. This term describes patients who meet general PD criteria, but do not fit into any category. Zimmerman et al. (2005) showed that in a large clinical sample, the unspecified group made up about 50% of the total. Verheul et al. (2007) found that patients with this diagnosis had a prevalence of 21% in a large clinical sample, and had serious deficits in psychosocial functioning.

For future research, unspecified PD is where the AMPD comes into its own. Patients who do not fit into traditional categories still need treatment, and clinical management could be guided by trait profiles rather than by traditional diagnostic systems.

A Biopsychosocial Model of Personality Disorders

A personality disorder is a complex condition, and no single factor accounts for its development. In a biopsychosocial (BPS) model, psychopathology emerges from multiple interactions between risk and protective factors (Engel, 1980). Personality disorder provides an excellent example. Biological, psychological, and social risk factors affect the development of personality, but none are sufficient to explain how traits become amplified to disorders. Thus only the cumulative and interactive effects of all these risk factors can explain how PDs develop.

Missing the Complexity of Personality Disorders

The BPS model is not routinely applied to PDs. There are many reasons why. One is that clinicians and researchers are trained in models that emphasize biology, psychology, or society. Moreover, PDs, in spite of the fact that they lead to disturbances in emotional regulation, behavior, and cognition that seriously affect functioning in work and relationships (Skodol et al., 2005), may not be considered in differential diagnosis. In both psychiatry and clinical psychology, the focus may fall on "comorbid" symptoms that accompany PDs, such as depression and anxiety, for which clinicians believe they have effective tools. In this way, the overarching construct of a PD is all too often missed.

Even when PDs are recognized, their clinical presentation may be viewed in the light of preexisting biases. Modern psychiatry, with its tendency to attribute symptoms to chemical imbalances and aberrant neurocircuitry, tends to see PD in a biological framework (New et al., 2008). This bias has been reinforced by the Research Domain Criteria (RDoC; Insel et al., 2010), which sees all of psychopathology as a biological problem that needs biological therapy.

Psychotherapists, who emphasize psychological causation, have favored the idea that childhood adversity accounts for the development of PDs (Bradley & Westen, 2005). However, this point of view fails to take into account the high rate of resilience in exposed children, as well as discordances between life histories and adult mental disorders (Paris, 2000). Only a few theorists (e.g., Millon, 1993) have seriously examined the possibility that cultural environments and social change are risk factors for PD.

Neither a strict biological model nor a narrow psychosocial perspective can do justice to the complexity of personality pathology. We need to go beyond linear thinking and develop an integrative, interactive conceptualization. Unfortunately, the human mind has difficulty dealing with complexity. We want the world to be univariate, even if it remains stubbornly multivariate.

Moreover, complex phenomena cannot be understood in a reductionistic framework. Mind is an emergent property of brain activity that cannot be explained at a neuronal level. The same principle applies to complex mental disorders. General systems theory (Sameroff, 1995) and stress-diathesis models (Monroe & Simons, 1991) view the pathways to disorder as multilevel and multidetermined. Unfortunately, this principle is not widely held in contemporary psychiatry, whose leaders prefer to follow the popular mantra that mental disorders are "nothing but" brain disorders (Insel et al., 2010).

Neuroscience has shed important light on psychopathology. Every mental disorder that has been studied is associated with some degree of genetic vulnerability. Yet genetic factors are not a predictable cause of any symptom, syndrome, or diagnosis. Rather, one sees interactions between multiple genes that mediate the development of symptoms, between genetic vulnerability and life experiences, as well as epigenetic mechanisms that mediate environmental influence on gene expression (Rutter, 2006).

The same complexities apply to understanding environmental risks. As confirmed by decades of research, no single adversity consistently leads to pathological sequelae. Rather, the risk lies in interactions between multiple adversities, whose cumulative effects are sufficient to convert risk to disorder (Rutter, 2006).

Moreover, interactions between diatheses and stressors are bidirectional. Genetic variability influences the way individuals respond to their environment, while environmental factors determine how genes are expressed. Cicchetti and Rogosch (1996) suggested that developmental psychopathology should respect two principles: *multifinality* (different outcomes can arise from similar risks) and *equifinality* (similar outcomes can arise from different risks).

Some experts have been critical of the BPS model for being eclectic rather than consistently interactional (Ghaemi, 2009). It is true that just piling on risk factors is not the best way to apply the model. It is also true that research needs to pay more attention to the precise measurement, and to measure interactions of each risk factor. However, rejecting the overall principles of BPS may just be a way of sticking to the perceived certainties of neuroscience, while avoiding the mind-boggling complexities of complex interactions.

To apply the principles of the BPS model to PDs, we can begin with the idea that the relationship between disorders, traits, and temperament is hierarchical and nested (Rutter, 1987). Heritable factors influence individual variability in temperament and traits, but are necessary (but not sufficient) causes of PDs.

By and large, trait variations are compatible with normality. They constitute vulnerabilities that only become maladaptive when amplified by life stressors. Thus while heritable factors account for close to half of individual variance in personality traits, the other half of the variance reflects environmental influences. Personality disorders develop when traits are amplified, leading to rigid and maladaptive ways of behaving, thinking, and feeling. Trait profiles determine what type of PD can develop.

While there is no definite boundary between traits and disorders, research on PDs shows that traits and symptoms measure different things and predict different things (Morey et al., 2007). Personality disorders are an amalgam of traits and symptoms. Some patients have few symptoms, as in narcissistic personality disorder (NPD) and obsessive compulsive personality disorder (OCPD). Others, such as borderline personality disorder (BPD), are associated with dramatic symptoms (such as cutting and repetitive overdosing) that are rarely seen in community populations. These symptoms are rooted in traits of impulsivity and affective instability (Crowell et al., 2009). When patients are followed over time, symptoms remit, but traits remain stable (Morey et al., 2007; Skodol et al., 2005). Thus, when patients no longer meet diagnostic criteria for a PD, they can still suffer dysfunction from problematic traits.

Genetic factors do not support the structure of PD clusters in the *Diagnostic and Statistical Manual of Mental Disorders* (DSM), Section II. Instead, in a multivariate twin study (Kendler et al., 2008), the authors (p. 1438) concluded:

Genetic risk factors for DSM-IV PDs do not reflect the cluster A, B, and C typology. Rather, 1 genetic factor reflects a broad vulnerability to PD pathology and/or negative emotionality. The 2 other genetic factors are more specific and reflect high impulsivity/low agreeableness and introversion. Unexpectedly, the cluster A, B, and C typology is well reflected in the structure of environmental risk factors, suggesting that environmental experiences may be responsible for the tendency of cluster A, B, and C PDs to co-occur.

Moreover, no molecular genetic findings have any specific association with personality traits or disorders. This situation is hardly unique in current research. Consistent biological markers have not been found for any form of psychopathology, as shown by genome-wide association studies (GWAS), complex syndromes are influenced by hundreds or thousands of different genes, and there are no consistent genetic markers for key diagnoses such as depression (Border et al., 2019).

A similar conclusion must be reached about biomarkers for PDs, i.e., that all findings are suggestive but sorely lacking in specificity and explanatory power. Thus, schizotypal PD is associated with abnormal eye-tracking that parallels schizophrenia (Siever & Davis, 1991). Borderline personality disorder can be associated with deficits in central serotonergic dysfunction (New et al., 2008). Functional magnetic resonance imaging (fMRI) shows that brain activity in BPD is consistent with emotion dysregulation (Donegan et al., 2003; Krause-Utz et al., 2014). There is evidence for reduction in prefrontal gray matter in psychopathic patients with antisocial personality disorder (ASPD), consistent with difficulty in controlling impulses and making judicious decisions (Glenn & Raine, 2008).

Yet at this point, these findings remain fragmentary. Much more sophisticated knowledge of how the brain works is needed to ground traits and disorders in biology. Plus, if personality is an emergent phenomenon, reflecting activity of the brain as a whole, these models may be of limited value.

Pathways from Traits to Disorders

Children are born with temperamental differences that lead to unique personalities. Even mental health professionals must have had the experience that, in spite of their best intentions, their children are simply not that malleable. The importance of temperament has been embodied in a witticism: "the mother of one child believes in the environment; the mother of two children believes in the genes".

These unique trait profiles can be the setting for either normality or psychopathology. Since temperament sets limits on the behavioral repertoire of children, stressors may not elicit new behaviors. Rather, negative experiences of any kind amplify already existing behavioral patterns. The process of amplification becomes stronger when stressors are chronic and enduring.

Many stressors amplify traits, but what the psychological risk factors for personality disorders all have in common is family dysfunction and inadequate parental care. Effective parenting requires an accommodation of parental strategies to the individual temperaments of children, i.e., "goodness of fit". When parents apply inflexible strategies, based more on their own needs than those of their children, unwanted traits in children, far from disappearing, are likely to be exaggerated.

Social factors become particularly important when dysfunction in the family is further amplified by dysfunction in the community. Breakdown of extended family ties, absence of a sense of community, normlessness related to the loss of consensual values, difficulty in developing social roles, problems in choosing an occupation and a partner, and the fragility of social networks, all constitute highly potent stressors. These effects are even more potent in individuals who are vulnerable by virtue of their trait profiles, and in those who also have dysfunctional families.

Let us consider as an example a dimension of personality that illustrates how all these factors interact. Extraversion is entirely adaptive under normal conditions; extraverted children are lively and social. In the presence of negative environmental factors, extraverts reach out to others for increased social contact. At some point, this trait could become exaggerated enough to become dysfunctional. For example, the child might demand to be the center of attention, and show protest behaviors when attention is withdrawn. These traits, when they lead consistently to inappropriate behaviors, eventually produce negative responses. When these same behaviors are used in many contexts, and are associated with conflictual interactions, they begin to correspond to the diagnostic criteria for PDs, such as the narcissistic type.

The other side of this trait is introversion. Being introverted is not necessarily associated with psychopathology, and children with this trait can be more self-sufficient. However, in the presence of environmental adversity, the introverted child may withdraw and seek greater protection from caretakers. When the environment is consistently negative, introversion can take on the characteristics of "anxious attachment". At a further level of amplification, these patterns may approximate the criteria for PDs in the anxious cluster (such as the dependent and avoidant categories).

Social factors can either amplify or reduce the intensity of personality traits. In modern societies, traits such as social anxiety that interfere with autonomous functioning are relatively more maladaptive, while narcissistic traits, which tend to interfere with social networks, but not with autonomous task performance, will be more adaptive. In a society where individualism is more important than collective values, the introvert is at greater risk (as one can see from the high prevalence of PDs associated with anxiety).

Interactions between Risk Factors

Let us now consider how the biological, psychological, and social factors in the personality disorders might interact. Biological and psychosocial risks create a feedback loop, in which abnormalities of temperament elicit negative responses. Others involve maladaptive personality traits that children and their families have in common. Still others consist of the effects of personality on the quality of life experiences, and how these experiences affect the individual.

Interactions between psychological and social factors involve indirect effects, such as the failure of the social environment to buffer negative psychological experiences. Others involve direct effects, in which a disintegrated social environment presents difficulties individuals with well-functioning families can master, but which are beyond the capacity of individuals coming from dysfunctional families.

If personality traits are alternative evolutionary strategies, more or less adaptive, depending on environmental demands, then the same environment could be positive for some individuals, while being a risk factor for others. It is when traits are discordant with social expectations that the risk for a personality disorder is greatest.

Biological variability, by itself, leads to individual differences in traits, not to personality disorders. Psychological factors, by themselves, also do not necessarily lead to personality disorders. Social factors, by themselves, represent stressors that everyone must live with. We need a biopsychosocial model, incorporating the interactions between all three factors, to explain the development of personality disorders.

One example of these interactions is the phenomenon of resilience. One of the most striking facts in developmental psychology is that most individuals exposed to negative experiences do not develop psychopathology. Those who fail to become disordered in spite of severe risks have been described as "resilient". The most likely explanations for this phenomenon are that resilience depends on adaptive personality traits, as well as on access to a buffering social environment.

Personality Disorders as Socially Sensitive

There is one more piece to be added to the model. Personality disorders are "socially sensitive" (Paris, 2004), in that they describe behaviors and emotions that can be shaped and molded by culture. Other disorders that can readily be described in this way include eating disorders and substance use disorders.

Personality disorders present with different symptoms in varying social contexts, and some categories might even be "culture-bound". The broad dimensions of personality are similar in different societies (McCrae & Terraciano, 2005), but there is definite cultural variation. A study of PDs across the world showed a very wide range of prevalence for categories and clusters across regions and countries (Huang et al., 2009). This finding underlines the role of sociocultural factors in determining symptoms.

Antisocial personality (and other impulsive spectrum disorders such as substance abuse) became more common in adolescents and young adults at the same time as increases in the prevalence of parasuicide and completed suicide in young people (Bland et al., 1998; Cash & Bridge, 2009). While the most recent data shows an increase of 30% in the suicide rate for all ages between 2000 and 2016 (Hedegaard et al., 2018), the rate for youth did not show the sharp spike seen in data from the 1960s. Nevertheless, since nearly a third of youth suicides can be diagnosed with BPD (Lesage et al., 1994), this represents a cohort effect.

This book argues that society is changing and that many young people can have difficulty adapting to these changes. Linehan (1993) hypothesized that patients with BPD have emotional dysregulation, and that decreases in social support in modern society amplify these traits by interfering with buffering mechanisms. This model, based on interactions between traits and psychosocial environments, is one of the most influential ideas today about the sources of BPD.

How Well Does the Model Account for Clinical Phenomena?

The model presented in this chapter can account for some of the essential characteristics of PDs. A high intensity of problematic temperamental characteristics interacts with the cumulative effects of multiple negative experiences during childhood. The chronic course of many PDs can be accounted for by a combination of the temporal stability of personality traits and feedback effects, in which maladaptive behaviors lead to negative consequences, which then further amplify traits.

The finding that the half of the environmental variance affecting personality traits is almost entirely "unshared" is one of the most surprising and important discoveries in the history of psychology. This data contradicts many classical theories in developmental and clinical psychology, which have focused on parenting as the main factor in personality development. However, that hypothesis is at best simplistic. The effects of life experience depend on gene–environment interactions. A child's temperament affects the response of other people in its environment, including family members. Another example is that even when the family provides a similar environment, every child perceives experiences differently and responds to them differently. Finally, many of the environmental factors affecting personality are extra-familial. Every child has important experiences with peers, with teachers, with community leaders, and with peer groups. All can be crucial for personality development.

This is not to dismiss the extensive body of evidence supporting the conclusion that childhood adversities are risk factors for PDs. However, a risk factor is not a cause. The presence of a risk factor does not mean that bad outcomes are inevitable, only that they are statistically more likely.

This model is also consistent with a vast literature on resilience to adversity. Even the most traumatic life events do not necessarily lead to psychopathology (Paris, 2000). Thus, only a minority of children exposed to childhood sexual abuse suffer measurable sequelae (Fergusson & Mullen, 1999). Those who are highly sensitive to their environment will be most likely to be affected, while those who are relatively insensitive may not (Belsky & Pluess, 2009).

When we see patients with traumatic histories, we are tempted to attribute their symptoms to these experiences. However, such conclusions fail to take into account the difference between patients, who are by definition affected by past adversities, and nonpatients, who may not be.

In summary, the relationship of early adversity to PD is statistical rather than predictive. Most children who are traumatized never develop PDs, and most patients with PDs have not been traumatized as children. Moreover, single traumatic events are rarely, by themselves, associated with pathological sequelae; continuously adverse circumstances have cumulative effects (Rutter, 1989). Repeated trauma can overwhelm temperamental resilience.

Finally, we have to remember that the relationship between adversity and PD assumes the validity of reports of life experiences occurring many years in the past. These memories are colored by recall bias, i.e., the tendency for those with symptoms in the present to remember more adversities in the past (Schacter, 1996). We need prospective studies to overcome this bias.

A good example of the kind of research is the Pittsburgh Girls Study (Stepp et al., 2016). In this community sample, children at risk were identified and have already been followed for several years into adolescence. What best predicted PD was a combination of symptoms in the child (disorders of behavioral control) along with high levels of conflict with mothers. This finding is highly consistent with a BPS or gene–environment model.

Psychotherapists who work with PD patients need to avoid routinely blaming families and consider abnormalities of temperament. It may well be true, however, that children who develop PDs need more support and attention from their parents than average. That is why one does always see the same pathology developing in siblings brought up in the same family.

To develop preventive programs for PDs, research would have to identify children at risk. Ideally, we would need to know which children are vulnerable, either because of temperamental variations or because of adverse circumstances, at an early age. Robins' (1966) classic follow-back study of conduct disorder showed that a childhood pattern of severe behavioral disturbance is a strong predictor of adult antisocial personality, but community samples with longitudinal follow-up have not collected a sufficient number of clinical cases to answer that question (Cohen et al., 2005).

Ten Principles for a Biopsychosocial Model of Personality Disorders

1. Personality disorders develop as amplifications of personality traits.
2. The early development and persistence of traits is best explained by biological factors.
3. Trait profiles are heritable, and determine which types of disorder can develop in any individual.
4. The biological risk factors for PDs consist of an unusual intensity of less adaptive traits, unbuffered by more adaptive traits.
5. Personality traits derive from interactions between temperament and social learning. However, temperament sets limits on the influence of learning and shapes the experiences to which individual are exposed.
6. Genetic factors account for about half the variance in traits, leaving another half for environmental influences that are unshared between children growing up in the same family.

7. Personality can develop relatively independent of parental input, and accounts for dramatic differences in personality characteristics between siblings raised in the same family.

8. Children with different temperamental dispositions respond to the same parental behaviors in different ways.

9. The social context outside the family shapes personality through behavioral expectations based on culture, either amplifying risks or supporting resilience.

10. Personality disorders are socially sensitive disorders, i.e., highly responsive to social demands and context.

Summary: An Integrative and Interactive Model

The biological, psychological, and social risk factors for personality disorders could be integrated within a single interactive and integrative model. Both genetic-temperamental and psychosocial factors would be necessary conditions for the development of personality disorders, but neither would be sufficient. A combination of risks (i.e., a "two-hit" or "multiple hit" mechanism) is required.

The effects of psychosocial adversity are greatest in individuals who are temperamentally predisposed to psychopathology. The cumulative effects of multiple risk factors, rather than single adversities, determines whether psychopathology develops. Finally, the specific disorder that emerges depends on temperamental profiles specific to the individual. All these mechanisms reflect gene–environment interactions. Abnormal temperament is associated with a greater sensitivity to environmental risk factors, and children with problematic temperaments are more likely to experience adversities (Rutter & Maughan, 1997). Vulnerable children elicit responses from others that tend to amplify their most problematic characteristics, creating a positive feedback loop. These adverse experiences further amplify traits, increasing the risk for further adverse experiences.

An integrative model can also account for the course of personality disorders over time (Paris, 2003). Early onset of pathology generally tends to reflect strongly abnormal temperament. By adolescence, when personality trait patterns become more stable, one can diagnose typical cases of personality disorder (with the exception of antisocial PD, which is required by DSM-5 to be called conduct disorder until age 18). In adult life, most personality disorders have a chronic course, but many patients improve with time (Skodol et al., 2005). Impulsive PDs are particularly likely to "burn out" by middle age (Paris, 2003).

An integrative model could have important implications for treatment. It would suggest that neither a strictly biological nor a purely psychosocial perspective is sufficient as a guide to effective therapy of PD. Moreover, neither a strictly biological perspective nor a strictly psychosocial perspective on PDs support either drugs or psychotherapy as the only or primary form of treatment. While maladaptive traits, established in childhood and reinforced during adult life, are difficult to change, the efficacy of psychotherapies in BPD has been supported by clinical trials (Paris, 2008).

Future research on PDs requires multiple perspectives. For the most part, biological researchers measure biological variables and psychosocial researchers measure psychosocial variables. Studies in which both aspects are assessed in the same sample with sophisticated measures are needed.

Once we obtain more knowledge concerning the diatheses and stressors driving both traits and disorders, we will be in a better position to develop more specific and more useful forms of treatment for these patients, more targeted biological interventions, more targeted forms of psychotherapy, as well as effective social interventions.

Chapter

10

Finding a Niche

The definition of a PD, an enduring pattern of dysfunction in work and intimate relationships, seems to point to chronicity. Yet we now know how to treat many of these patients successfully. Some of the protective factors that increase or decrease risk are similar to what effective therapy can accomplish.

This chapter will discuss how to help patients find a niche in life, establish a social network, and increase their "social capital" (see definition below). People differ in how good they are accomplishing these goals. Those who are better at making connections will be less vulnerable to PDs and recover from them more readily.

It is important to find a social niche that fits the individual's personality trait profile. This is generally found by working and/or studying. I am only one of several experts who emphasize this aspect of recovery, and ask patients to do their part of the treatment by "getting a life" (Zanarini, 2005). That usually means establishing a direction and a commitment to a social role through an occupation. Tyrer and Tyrer (2018) call this approach to treatment "nidotherapy", i.e., finding a niche.

By and large, patients who are chronically unemployed and socially isolated will benefit little from therapy. Treatment is rather like taking a lecture course with no lab or reading list. It is no use learning how to control emotions and impulses if there is no place to apply these skills. Patients with PDs need to ground themselves in places in the occupational and social world that are appropriate to their characteristics. Treatment can help them to find that niche.

Many PD patients we see make the mistake of trying to find another person to provide them with an identity, but you cannot expect to be loved without first becoming a person in your own right. You also have to be someone to love someone.

Since I work with young patients, most of whom have borderline personality disorder (BPD), this can mean encouraging patients recovering from a breakup to take a break from intimacy. They need to build up a sense of self, which is not something you can just decide to have. Self-esteem derives not from narcissistic entitlement, but from real accomplishments and commitments in the world. Our program therefore tells patients they have to set a goal of either working or studying to prepare for work and to accomplish that during the treatment.

What about patients who are older, chronically unemployed, and socially isolated? In such cases, therapeutic sights have to be set much lower. Some of these patients can get involved with volunteer work or community organizations. The main thing is what cognitive behavioral therapy (CBT) calls behavioral activation (Jacobson et al., 1996). In simple terms, there is nothing worse for recovery than sitting at home all day watching TV.

The Role of Social Capital in Treatment

The term "social capital" was introduced by the French sociologist Pierre Bourdieu (1986). Similar ideas had previously been described in the sociological literature (Hanifan, 1916; Jacobs, 1961).

Social capital can be understood as describing links between people that are based on membership in a group and on common interests, rather than on kinship (Almedon, 2005; Woolcock, 1998). The construct can be divided into mechanisms of bonding within the same community, or of bridging across communities (Dolfsma & Dannreuther, 2003). Higher levels of social capital are associated with mental health and recovery from mental illness (Tew et al., 2011).

The key to this idea is that, like other forms of investment, social capital should be spread out so that if one stock fails, the social portfolio does not go bankrupt. Therefore, it is wise not to have a single investment, in a relationship or in a job, but a balanced portfolio. This is where BPD patients run into trouble when their significant other is "my everything". It is also where obsessive compulsive personality disorder (OCPD) patients have difficulty if their identity is totally tied up in their work. Instead, it is more useful to have group of friends, colleagues, and acquaintances, each of which provides something different. Social capital can therefore be accumulated and bear psychological "interest" by being available when times are tough.

There is a crucial difference between social networks and intimate relationships. It is important to accumulate *all* kind of connections, from intimate to casual. This can be thought of as a wise investment strategy. Having friends and being attached to a community can provide these commitments. The more people we have in our lives, the less is the risk that losing one investment will cause emotional bankruptcy.

Moreover, relationships of any kind, by themselves, are insufficient to establish a secure and balanced account of social capital. In this light, you cannot get a life without looking for a job. Work provides a social role, promotes a sense of the future, and offers attachments of a different kind. Chronic unemployment provides none of these things. This is why many programs expect PD patients to get a job or to go to school to prepare for one.

The construct of social capital was brought to the attention of the educated public by the American political scientist Robert Putnam (2000). Putnam applied scales specifically developed to measure the construct (Burdine et al., 1999), and found evidence for its overall decline in modern American society. A relative decline of social capital may also now be a worldwide trend, given the rapid growth of urbanization and globalization (McKenzie, 2008).

Social capital means that people are connected and have some form of generalized trust (Giordano & Lindström, 2011). In contrast, in a society in which traditional family and community structures have weakened, and in which individuals focus more on self and less on others (Markus & Kitayama, 1994), trust becomes more difficult.

Social capital has a positive association with mental health (Almedon, 2005; Lofors & Sundquist, 2007; McKenzie & Harpham, 2006) and to physical health (Kawachi et al., 2007; Song, 2011). Since it enhances recovery from mental illness (Tew et al., 2011), the term "recovery capital" has been used (Tew, 2012). However, we lack data to show that any specific intervention increases social capital in patients (De Silva et al., 2005; McKenzie et al., 2002).

Much research on social capital has focused on patients with severe mental illness and/or immigrant populations (McKenzie et al., 2002). The construct has also been applied to common mental disorders (De Silva et al., 2005). Up to now, it has not been studied in PDs. Nevertheless, one can hypothesize that the prevalence of PDs is affected by levels of social capital in the community, and the ability of people to make use of it.

Social Capital and Recovery from Personality Disorders

One of the fundamental problems in PD patients derives from deficits in social skills, leading to weak social networks and social support (Rey et al., 1997). These difficulties have an impact on outcome: many patients with PDs, when followed for 10 years, lose active symptoms but continue to have serious psychosocial dysfunction (Gunderson et al., 2011; Zanarini et al., 2012).

These deficits (lack of social roles, few friends, failure to participate in community activities) constitute a lack of social capital. Long-term follow-up shows that patients generally do better when involved in their community through work, interest groups, religious affiliation, voluntary work, or voluntary organizations (Paris & Zweig-Frank, 2001).

Interventions for PD could be developed that have specific effects on social capital. Currently, none of the treatment packages for evidence-based therapies focus on social integration. They offer an effective combination of group and individual therapy designed to control acute symptoms, although increased social capital is an implicit goal. Even when recovered, many PD patients make heavy use of services (Hörz et al., 2010). The fact that most patients with BPD continue to experience psychosocial deficits led Gunderson and Links (2008) to recommend that they should almost always be encouraged to seek work and/or further education. Zanarini (2005) has called for the development of active rehabilitation programs.

It is counterproductive to accept that PD patients should become or remain dependent on long-term medical disability. To "get a life" these patients need to return to the workforce. Setting these goals is particularly relevant for younger patients, who have more time and more options. Even in patients who are unlikely to find gainful employment, rehabilitation programs can build social capital through volunteer work and commitments to community organizations.

Tyrer and Tyrer's (2018) "nidotherapy" applies the principles of social psychiatry to PDs, harmonizing environmental niches with personality traits. The aim is to find social roles that fit the needs of patients with trait profiles ranging from emotional instability to overconscientiousness. This approach makes a good deal of sense, and has been tested in clinical trials (Ranger et al., 2009; Tyrer et al., 2011b, 2017).

It should be kept in mind that patients with PDs are not always ready to follow recommendations for rehabilitation. They may provide their therapists with reasons why doing so is unwise or impossible – the job market is poor and friendships have always proved disappointing. Changes that increase social capital require motivation, and for some people, isolation is the least risky alternative. Yet even in the most dysfunctional patients, incremental change is possible.

Rehabilitation models have been widely researched in patients with psychoses (Vaddadi, 2010), who often function on the margins of society and need highly structured interventions. However, in PD, research shows that most patients find employment on their own, even when social networks are marginal (Gunderson et al., 2011). Even those who remain seriously disabled may still be able to find social roles as volunteers. They can be guided to find social capital on more neutral ground, in which dependency and conflict are less likely to emerge. By and large, this population can be encouraged to stay off welfare, to continue their education, to join community organizations, and to maintain whatever social networks they have.

Conclusions

We do not need a new form of therapy for personality disorders, but can combine the best ideas from existing methods (Livesley, 2012). Social capital remains a missing element: changing cognitions in the present can only be effective if there is a proper environment to apply them. It is possible that advocacy for the mentally ill could open up more of these options. Nevertheless, even within current constraints, intervention can be helpful.

In summary, many patients with personality disorders suffer from not getting a life (Zanarini, 2005). Mental health professionals need to encourage them to finding a niche in society that provides some degree of involvement and social status.

References

Achenbach, T. M., & McConaughy, S. H. (1997). *Empirically based assessment of child and adolescent psychopathology: Practical applications* (2nd ed.). Thousand Oaks, CA: Sage.

Ackerman, R. A., Witt, E. A., Donnellan, M. B., Trzesniewski, K. H., Robins, R. W., & Kashy, D. A. (2011). What does the Narcissistic Personality Inventory really measure? *Assessment, 18*, 67–87.

Alarcón, R. D., Becker, A. E., Lewis-Fernandez, R., Like, R. C., Desai, P., Foulks, E., & Primm, A. (2009). Issues for DSM-V: The role of culture in psychiatric diagnosis. *Journal of Nervous and Mental Disease, 197*, 559–660.

Alarcón, R. D., Foulks, E. F., & Vakkur, M. (1998). *Culture and personality disorders*. New York, NY: John Wiley & Sons.

Almedon, A. M. (2005). Social capital and mental health: An interdisciplinary review of primary evidence. *Social Science & Medicine, 61*, 943–964.

Amato, P. R., Booth, A., Johnson, D. R., & Rogers, S. J. (2009). *Alone together: How marriage in America is changing*. Cambridge, MA: Harvard University Press.

American Psychiatric Association. (1952). *Diagnostic and statistical manual of mental disorders*. Washington, DC: American Psychiatric Press.

(1968). *Diagnostic and statistical manual of mental disorders* (2nd ed.). Washington, DC: American Psychiatric Press.

(1980). *Diagnostic and statistical manual of mental disorders* (3rd ed.). Washington, DC: American Psychiatric Press.

(2013). *Diagnostic and statistical manual of mental disorders* (5th ed.). Washington, DC: American Psychiatric Press.

Arbel, N., & Stravynski, A. (1991). A retrospective study of separation in the development of adult avoidant personality disorder. *Acta Psychiatrica Scandinavica, 83*, 174–178.

Asmolov, G. (2016). Psychology of modernity as a social situation of development: Challenges of uncertainty, complexity and diversity. *Procedia – Social and Behavioral Sciences, 233*, 27–34.

Bandura, A. (1977). *Social learning theory*. Englewood Cliffs, NJ: Prentice Hall.

Barkow, J. H., Cosmides, L., & Tooby, J. (1992). *The adapted mind: Evolutionary psychology and the generation of culture*. New York, NY: Oxford University Press.

Bateman, A., & Fonagy, P. (2004). *Psychotherapy for borderline personality disorder: Mentalization based treatment*. Oxford, UK: Oxford University Press.

Baudry, L. (1986). *The frenzy of renown: Fame and its history*. New York, NY: Vintage.

Baumeister, R. F., & Leary, M. R. (1995). Desire for interpersonal attachments as a fundamental human motivation. *Psychological Bulletin, 117*, 497–529.

Beck, A. T., & Freeman, A. (2015). *Cognitive therapy of personality disorders* (2nd ed.). New York, NY: Guilford.

Bellah, R. N., Madsen, R., Sullivan, W. M., Swidler, A., & Tipton, S. M. (1985). *Habits of the heart.* Berkeley, CA: University of California Press.

Belsky, J., & Cassidy, J. (1994). Attachment: Theory and evidence. In M. Rutter & D. Hay (Eds.), *Development through life: A handbook for clinicians* (pp. 373–402). Oxford, UK: Blackwell.

Belsky, J., & Pluess, M. (2009). The nature (and nurture?) of plasticity in early human development. *Perspectives in Psychological Science, 4*, 345–351.

Berrios, G. E. (1993). European views on personality disorders: A conceptual history. *Comprehensive Psychiatry, 34*, 14–30.

Black, D. W. (2008). *Bad boys, bad men: Confronting antisocial personality disorder (sociopathy)* (2nd ed.). New York, NY: Oxford University Press.

(2015). The natural history of antisocial personality disorder. *Canadian Journal of Psychiatry, 60*, 309–314.

Blackmore, S. (1999). *The meme machine.* Oxford, UK: Oxford University Press.

Bland, R. C., Dyck, R. J., Newman, S. C., & Orn, H. (1998). Attempted suicide in Edmonton. In A. A. Leenaars, S. Wenckstern, I. Sakinofsky, R. J. Dyck, M. J. Kral, & R. C. Bland (Eds.), *Suicide in Canada* (pp. 136–150). Toronto: University of Toronto Press.

Border, R., Johnson, E. C., Evans, L. M., Smolen, L. M., Berley, N., Sullivan, P. F., & Keller, M. C. (2019). No support for historical candidate gene or candidate gene-by-interaction hypotheses for major depression across multiple large samples. *American Journal of Psychiatry, 176*, 376–387.

Bornstein, R. (2005). *The dependent patient: A practitioner's guide.* Washington, DC: American Psychological Association.

Bouchard, T. J. Jr., Lykken, D. T., McGue, M., Segal, N. L., & Tellegen, A. (1990). Sources of human psychological differences: The Minnesota study of twins reared apart. *Science, 250*, 223–228.

Bourdieu, P. (1986). The forms of capital. In J. E. Richardson (Ed.), *Handbook of theory of research for the sociology of education* (pp. 46–58). Westport, CT: Greenwood Press.

Bowlby, J. (1969). *Attachment.* London: Hogarth Press.

Bradley, R., & Westen, D. (2005). The psychodynamics of borderline personality disorder: A view from developmental psychopathology. *Development and Psychopathology, 17*, 927–957.

Briley, D. A., & Tucker-Drob, E. M. (2014). Genetic and environmental continuity in personality development: A meta-analysis. *Psychological Bulletin, 140*, 1303–1331.

Brown, G., & Harris, T. (1978). *Social origins of depression.* London: Tavistock.

Brown, M. Z., Comtois, K. A., & Linehan, M. M. (2002). Reasons for suicide attempts and nonsuicidal self-injury in women with borderline personality disorder. *Journal of Abnormal Psychology, 111,* 198–202.

Browne, A., & Finkelhor, D. (1986). Impact of child sexual abuse: A review of the literature. *Psychological Bulletin, 99,* 66–77.

Burdine, J. N., Felix, M., Wallerstein, N., Abel, A. L., Wiltrait, C. J., & Musselman, Y. J. (1999). Measurement of social capital. *Annals of the New York Academy of Sciences, 25,* 393–395.

Butcher, J. N. (2010). Personality assessment from the nineteenth to the early twenty-first century: Past achievements and contemporary challenges. *Annual Review of Clinical Psychology, 6,* 1–20.

Button, T. M. M., Scourfield, J., Martin, N., Purcell, S., & McGuffin, P. (2005). Family dysfunction interacts with genes in the causation of antisocial symptoms. *Behavior Genetics, 35,* 115–120.

Cain, N. M., Pincus, A. L., & Ansell, E. B. (2008). Narcissism at the crossroads: Phenotypic description of pathological narcissism across clinical theory, social/personality psychology, and psychiatric diagnosis. *Clinical Psychology Review, 4,* 638–656.

Caldwell-Harris, C. L., & Aycicegi, A. (2006). When personality and culture clash: The psychological distress of allocentrics in an individualist culture and idiocentrics in a collectivist culture. *Transcultural Psychiatry, 43,* 331–361.

Campbell, W. K., & Miller, J. D. (Eds.). (2011). *Handbook of narcissism and narcissistic personality disorder.* New York, NY: Wiley.

Campbell, W. K., Miller, J. D., & Buffardi, L. E. (2010). The United States and the "culture of narcissism": An examination of perceptions of national character. *Social Psychological and Personality Science, 1,* 222–229.

Cantor-Graae, E., & Selten, J. P. (2005). Schizophrenia and migration: A meta-analysis and review. *American Journal of Psychiatry, 162,* 12–24.

Cash, S. J., & Bridge, J. A. (2009). Epidemiology of youth suicide and suicidal behavior. *Current Opinion in Pediatrics, 21,* 613–619.

Caspi, A., Moffitt, T. E., Newman, D. L., & Silva, P. A. (1996). Behavioral observations at age three predict adult psychiatric disorders: Longitudinal evidence from a birth cohort. *Archives of General Psychiatry, 53,* 1033–1039.

Cassidy, J., & Shaver, P. R. (2018). *Handbook of attachment: Theory, research, and clinical applications* (3rd ed.). New York, NY: Guilford.

Cavalli-Sforza, L. L., Feldman, M. W., Chen, K.-h., & Dornbusch, S. M. (1982). Theory and observation in cultural transmission. *Science, 218* (4567), 19–27.

Chagnon, N. A. (1988). Life histories, blood revenge, and warfare in a tribal population. *Science, 239* (4843), 985–992.

Charron, M. F. (1981). *Le suicide au Québec.* Québec, Ministère des Affaires Sociales, Gouvernement du Québec.

Cicchetti, D., & Rogosch, F. A. (1996). Equifinality and multifinality in developmental psychopathology. *Development and Psychopathology, 8,* 597–600.

Cleckley, H. (1976). *The mask of sanity* (5th ed.). New York, NY: Mosby.

Cohen, P., & Cohen, J. (1984). The clinician's illusion. *Archives of General Psychiatry, 41,* 1178–1182.

Cohen, P., Crawford, T. N., Johnson, J. G., & Kasen, S. (2005). The children in the community study of developmental course of personality disorder. *Journal of Personality Disorders, 19,* 466–486.

Coid, J., Yang, M., Tyrer, P., Roberts, A., & Ullrich, S. (2006). Prevalence and correlates of personality disorder in Great Britain. *British Journal of Psychiatry, 188,* 423–431.

Coid, J. W., & Ullrich, S. (2010). Antisocial personality disorder is on a continuum with psychopathy. *Comprehensive Psychiatry, 51,* 426–433.

Compton, W. M., Helzer, J., Hwu, H. G., & Yeh, E. K. (1991). New methods in cross-cultural psychiatry: Psychiatric illness in Taiwan and the United States. *American Journal of Psychiatry, 148,* 1697–1704.

Costa, P. T., & Widiger, T. A. (2013). *Personality disorders and the five factor model of personality* (3rd ed.). Washington, DC: American Psychological Association.

Craker, N., & March, N. (2016). The dark side of Facebook®: The Dark Tetrad, negative social potency, and trolling behaviours. *Personality and Individual Differences, 102,* 79–84.

Crawford, M., Sanatinia, R., Barrett, B. M., Cunningham, G., Dale, O., Ganguli, P., Lawrence-Smith, G., Leeson, V., Lemonsky, F., Lykomitrou, G., Montgomery, A. A., Morriss, R., Munjiza, J., Paton, C., Skorodzien, I., Singh, V., Tan, W., Tyrer, P., Reilly, J. G., & LABILE study team. (2018). The clinical effectiveness and cost-effectiveness of lamotrigine in borderline personality disorder: A randomized placebo-controlled trial. *American Journal of Psychiatry, 175,* 756–764.

Crawford, T. N., Livesley, W. J., Jang, K. L., Shaver, P. R., Cohen, P., & Ganiban, J. (2007). Insecure attachment and personality disorder: A twin study of adults. *European Journal of Personality, 21,* 191–208.

Cristea, I. A., Gentilla, C., Cotet, C. D., Palomba, D., Barbui, C., & Cuijpers, P. (2017). Efficacy of psychotherapies for borderline personality disorder: A systematic review and meta-analysis. *JAMA Psychiatry, 74,* 319–328.

Crowe, R. R. (1974). An adoption study of antisocial personality. *Archives of General Psychiatry, 31,* 785–791.

Crowell, S. E., Beauchaine, T., & Linehan, M. M. (2009). A biosocial developmental model of borderline personality: Elaborating and extending Linehan's theory. *Psychological Bulletin, 135,* 495–510.

Curtin, S. C., Warner, M., & Hedegaard, H. (2016). *Increase in suicide in the United States 1999–2014.* Washington, DC: National Center for Health Statistics, Brief #241, April.

Cushman, P. (1990). *Constructing the self, constructing America: A cultural history of psychotherapy.* New York, NY: Addison-Wesley.

Dawkins, R. (1976). *The selfish gene.* Oxford, UK: Oxford University Press.

De Brito, S., & Hodgins, S. (2009). Antisocial personality disorder. In M. McMurran & R. Howard (Eds.), *Personality, personality disorder, and* violence: An evidence-based approach (pp. 133–155). London: John Wiley.

De Silva, M. J., McKenzie, K., Harpham, T., & Huttly, S. (2005). Social capital and mental illness: A systematic review. *Journal of Epidemiology and Community Health, 59*, 619–627.

Deci, E. L., & Ryan, R. M. (2002). *Handbook of self-determination research*. Rochester, NY: University of Rochester Press.

Degenhardt, K., Stockings, E., Patton, G., Hall, W. S., & Linskey, M. (2016). The increasing global health priority of substance use in young people. *Lancet Psychiatry, 3*, 251–264.

DeMause, L. (Ed.). (1974). *The history of childhood*. New York, NY: Psychohistory Press.

DeWall, C. N., Pond, R. S., Campbell, W. K., & Twenge, J. (2011). Tuning in to psychological change: Linguistic markers of psychological traits and emotions over time in popular U.S. song lyrics. *Psychology of Aesthetics, Creativity, and the Arts, 5*, 200–207.

Dhawan, N., Kunik, M. E., Oldham, J., & Coverdale, J. (2010). Prevalence and treatment of narcissistic personality disorder in the community: A systematic review. *Comprehensive Psychiatry, 54*, 333–339.

Dohrenwend, B. P., & Dohrenwend, B. S. (1969). *Social status and psychological disorder: A causal inquiry*. New York, NY: Wiley.

Dolan, B., & Coid, J. (1993). *Psychopathic and antisocial personality disorders: Treatment and research issues*. London: Gaskell/Royal College of Psychiatrists.

Dolan, M., & Park, I. (2002). The neuropsychology of antisocial personality disorder. *Psychological Medicine, 32*, 417–442.

Dolfsma, W., & Dannreuther, C. (2003). Subjects and boundaries: Contesting social capital-based policies. *Journal of Economic Issues, 37*, 405–413.

Donegan, N. H., Sanislow, C. A., Blumberg, H. P., Fulbright, R. K., Lacadie. C., & Skudlarski, P. (2003). Amygdala hyperreactivity in borderline personality disorder: Implications for emotional dysregulation. *Biological Psychiatry, 54*, 1284–1293.

Donnellan, M. B., Trzesniewski, K. H., & Robins, R. W. (2009). An emerging epidemic of narcissism or much ado about nothing? *Journal of Research in Personality, 43*, 498–501.

Durham, W. H. (1992). *Co-evolution: Genes, culture, and human diversity*. Stanford, CA: Stanford University Press.

Durkheim, E. (1897/1997). *Suicide*. New York, NY: Free Press.

Durvasula, S., Lysonski, S., & Watson, J. (2001). Does vanity describe other cultures? A cross-cultural examination of the vanity scale. *Journal of Consumer Affairs, 35*, 180–199.

Easterlin, R. (2015). Happiness and economic growth – the evidence. In W. Glatzer, L. Canfield, V. Mailer, & M. Rojas (Eds.), *Global handbook of quality of life* (pp. 283–299). New York, NY: Oxford University Press.

Eaton, N. R., South, S. C., & Krueger, R. F. (2010). The meaning of comorbidity among common mental disorders. In T. Millon, R. Krueger, & E. Simonsen (Eds.), *Contemporary directions in psychopathology: Scientific foundations of the DSM-V and ICD-11* (pp. 223–241). New York, NY: Guilford.

Eid, M., & Diener, E. (2001). Norms for experiencing emotions in different cultures: Inter- and intranational differences. *Journal of Personality and Social Psychology, 81,* 869–885.

Eisenberg, L. (1986). Mindless and brainless in psychiatry. *British Journal of Psychiatry, 148,* 497–508.
(1995). The social construction of the human brain. *American Journal of Psychiatry, 152,* 1563–1575.

Engel, G. L. (1980). The clinical application of the biopsychosocial model. *American Journal of Psychiatry, 137,* 535–544.

Erikson, E. (1950). *Childhood and society.* New York, NY: Norton.

Etzioni, A. (1993). *The spirit of community: Rights, responsibilities and the communitarian agenda.* New York, NY: Crown.

Eysenck, H. J. (1982). Culture and personality abnormalities. In I. Al-Issa (Ed.), *Culture and psychopathology* (pp. 277–308). Baltimore, MD: University Park Press.

Eysenck, H. J., & Gudjonsson, G. H. (1989). *The causes and cures of criminality.* New York, NY: Plenum Press.

Farrell, G., Tilley, N., & Tseloni, A. (2014). Why the crime drop? *Crime and Justice, 43,* 421–490.

Farrington, D. P. (1993). Childhood origins of teenage antisocial behaviour and adult social dysfunction. *Journal of the Royal Society of Medicine, 86,* 13–17.

Farrington, D. P., & Welsh, B. C. (2008). *Saving children from a life of crime: Early risk factors and effective intervention.* Oxford, UK: Oxford University Press.

Fava, M. (2003). Diagnosis and definition of treatment-resistant depression. *Biological Psychiatry, 53,* 649–659.

Favazza, A. (1987). *Bodies under siege: Self-mutilation in culture and psychiatry.* Baltimore, MD: Johns Hopkins University Press.

Fergusson, D. M., & Mullen, P. E. (1999). *Childhood sexual abuse: An evidence based perspective.* Thousand Oaks, CA: Sage Publications.

Finkelhor, D., & Jones, L. (2006). Why have child maltreatment and child victimization declined? *Journal of Social Issues, 62,* 685–716.

Finkelhor, D., Ormrod, R. K., Turner, H. A., & Hamby, S. L. (2005). The victimization of children and youth: A comprehensive, national survey. *Child Maltreatment, 10,* 5–25.

Finkelhor, D., Turner, H. A., Shattuck, A. M., & Hamby, S. L. (2013). Violence, crime, and abuse exposure in a national sample of children and youth. *JAMA Pediatrics, 167,* 614–621.

Finkelhor, D., Vanderminden, J., Turner, H., Hamby, S., & Shattuuck, A. (2014). Child maltreatment rates assessed in a national household survey of caregivers and youth. *Child Abuse and Neglect, 38,* 1421–1435.

Fischer, C. (2010). *Made in America.* Chicago: University of Chicago Press.

Fok, M. L. Y., Stewart, R., Hayes, R. D., & Moran, P. (2014). Predictors of natural and unnatural mortality among patients with personality disorder: Evidence from a large UK case register. *PLoS ONE, 9,* e100979.

Forman, E. M., Berk, M. S., Henriques, G. R., Brown, G. K., & Beck, A. T. (2004). History of multiple suicide attempts as a behavioral marker of severe psychopathology. *American Journal of Psychiatry, 161,* 437–443.

Foster, J. D., Campbell, W. K., & Twenge, J. M. (2003). Individual differences in narcissism: Inflated self-views across the lifespan and around the world. *Journal of Research in Personality, 37,* 469–486.

Freeman, A., Tyrovolas, S., & Koyanag, A. (2016). The role of socio-economic status in depression: Results from the COURAGE aging survey in Europe. *BMC Public Health, 16,* 1098.

Fromm, E. (1955). *The sane society.* New York, NY: Holt, Rinehardt, Winston.

Furedi, F. (2004). *Therapy culture: Cultivating vulnerability in an uncertain age.* London: Routledge.

Furstenberg, F. F. (2000). The sociology of adolescence and youth in the 1990s: A critical commentary. *Journal of Marriage and the Family, 62,* 896–910.

Gellner, E. (1993). *The psychoanalytic movement* (2nd ed.). London: Fontana.

Ghaemie, S. N. (2009). The rise and fall of the biopsychosocial model. *British Journal of Psychiatry, 195,* 3–4.

Giddens, A. (1991). *The consequences of modernity.* Stanford, CA: Stanford University Press.

Giordano, G. N., & Lindström, M. (2010). The impact of changes in different aspects of social capital and material conditions on self-rated health over time: A longitudinal cohort study. *Social Science and Medicine, 70,* 700–710.

(2011). Social capital and change in psychological health over time. *Social Science & Medicine, 72,* 1219–1227.

Glenn, A. L., & Raine, A. (2008). The neurobiology of psychopathy. *Psychiatric Clinics North America, 31,* 463–475.

Goldberg, E. M., & Morrison, S. L. (1988). Schizophrenia and social class. In C. Buck et al. (Eds.), *The challenge of epidemiology: Issues and selected readings* (pp. 368–383). Washington, DC: Pan American Health Organization.

Gone, J. P., & Kirmayer, L. J. (2010). On the wisdom of considering culture and context in psychopathology. In T. Millon, R. Krueger, & E. Simonsen (Eds.), *Contemporary directions in psychopathology: Scientific foundations of the DSM-V and ICD-11* (pp. 72–96). New York, NY: Guilford.

Gordon, R. A. (1990). *Anorexia and bulimia.* Cambridge, MA: Blackwell.

Graff, H., & Mallin, K. R. (1967). The syndrome of the wrist cutter. *American Journal of Psychiatry, 146,* 789–790.

Gramlich, J. (2019). 5 facts about crime in the USA. Pew Research Center. org, accessed August 19, 2019.

Grant, B. F. (1997). Prevalence and correlates of alcohol use and DSM-IV alcohol dependence in the United States: Results of the National Longitudinal Alcohol Epidemiologic Survey. *Journal of Studies on Alcohol, 58,* 464–473.

Grant, B. F., Hasin, D. S., Stinson, F. S., Dawson, D. A., Chou, S. P., & Ruan, W. J. (2004). Prevalence, correlates, and disability of personality disorders in the United States: Results from the National Epidemiologic Survey on Alcohol and Related Conditions. *Journal of Clinical Psychiatry, 65,* 948–958.

Gunderson, J. G., & Links, P. (2008). *Borderline personality disorder: A clinical guide* (2nd ed.). Washington, DC: American Psychiatric Press.

Gunderson, J. G., & Phillips, K. A. (1991). A current view of the interface between borderline personality disorder and depression. *American Journal of Psychiatry, 148*, 967–975.

Gunderson, J. G., & Singer, M. T. (1975). Defining borderline patients: An overview. *American Journal of Psychiatry, 132*, 1–9.

Gunderson, J. G., Stout, R. L., McGlashan, T. H., Shea, M. T., Morey, L. C., Grilo, C. M., Zanarini, M. C., Yen, S., Markowitz, J. C., Sanislow, C., Ansell, E., Pinto, A., & Skodol, A. E. (2011). Ten-year course of borderline personality disorder: Psychopathology and function from the Collaborative Longitudinal Personality Disorders Study. *Archives of General Psychiatry, 68*, 827–837.

Gupta, S., & Mattoo, S. K. (2012). Personality disorders: Prevalence and demography at a psychiatric outpatient in North India. *International Journal of Social Psychiatry, 58*, 146–152.

Hale, R. (1995). *The rise and crisis of psychoanalysis in the United States.* New York, NY: Oxford University Press.

Hanifan, L. J. (1916). The rural school community center. *Annals of the American Academy of Political and Social Science, 67*, 130–138.

Hare, R. D. (2003). *Manual for the revised psychopathy checklist* (2nd ed.). Toronto: Multi-Health Systems.

Harris, J. R. (1998). *The nurture assumption.* New York, NY: Free Press.

Hart, S. D., & Hare, R. D. (1996). Psychopathy and antisocial personality disorder. *Current Opinion in Psychiatry, 9*, 129–132.

Hechtman, L. (Ed.). (2016). *Attention deficit hyperactivity disorder: Adult outcome and its predictor.* New York, NY: Oxford University Press.

Hedegaard, H., Curtin, S. C., & Warner, M. (2018). Suicide rates in the United States continue to increase. NCHS Data Brief No. 309. National Center for Health Statistics. www.cdc.gov/nchs/products/databriefs/db309.htm

Helzer, J. E., & Canino, G. J. (Eds.). (1992). *Alcoholism in North America, Europe, and Asia.* New York, NY: Oxford University Press.

Hermann, A. D., Brunell, A. B., & Foster, J. D. (Eds.). (2018). *Handbook of trait narcissism: Key advances, research methods and controversies.* New York, NY: Springer.

Hetherington, E. M., Cox, M., & Cox, R. (1985). Long-term effects of divorce and remarriage on the adjustment of children. *Journal of the American Academy of Child Psychiatry, 24*, 518–530.

Hidaka, B. H. (2012). Depression as a disease of modernity: Explanations for increasing prevalence. *Journal of Affective Disorders, 140*, 205–214.

Hill, P. L., & Roberts, B. W. (2011). Examining "developmental me": A review of narcissism in a life span perspective. In W. K. Campbell & J. Miller (Eds.), *Handbook of narcissism and narcissistic personality disorder* (pp. 191–201). New York, NY: Wiley.

Horney, K. (1940). *The neurotic personality of our time.* New York, NY: Norton.

Horton, R. S. (2011). Parenting and narcissism. In W. K. Campbell & J. Miller (Eds.), *Handbook of narcissism and narcissistic personality disorder* (pp. 181–190). New York, NY: Wiley.

Horton, R. S., Bleau, G., & Drwecki, D. (2006). Parenting Narcissus: What are the links between parenting and narcissism? *Journal of Personality, 74,* 345–352.

Horwitz, A. V. (2002). *Creating mental illness.* Chicago: University of Chicago Press.

Hörz, S., Zanarini, M. C., Frankenburg, F. R., Reich, D. B., & Fitzmaurice, G. (2010). Ten-year use of mental health services by patients with borderline personality disorder and with other Axis II disorders. *Psychiatric Services, 61,* 612–616.

Huang, Y., Kotov, R., de Girolamo, G., Preti, A., Angermeyer, M., Benjet, C., Demyttenaere, K., Graaf, R., Gureje, O., Nasser Karam, A., Lee, S., Lépine, J. P., Matschinger, H., Posada-Villa, J., Suliman, S., Vilagut, S., & Kessler, R. C. (2009). DSM–IV personality disorders in the WHO World Mental Health Surveys. *British Journal of Psychiatry, 195,* 46–53.

Hudson, C. G. (2005). Socioeconomic status and mental illness: Tests of the social causation and selection hypotheses. *American Journal of Orthopsychiatry, 75,* 3–18.

Hurst, C. E. (2007). *Social inequality: Forms, causes, and consequences* (6th ed.). Boston: Pearson Education.

Hwu, H. G., Yeh, E. K., & Change, L. Y. (1989). Prevalence of psychiatric disorders in Taiwan defined by the Chinese Diagnostic Interview Schedule. *Acta Psychiatrica Scandinavica, 79,* 136–147.

Inkeles, A., & Smith, D. H. (1974). *Becoming modern: Individual change in six developing countries.* Cambridge, MA: Harvard University Press.

Insel, T., Cuthbert, B., Garvey, M., Heinssen, R., Pine, D. S., Quinn, K., Sanislow, C., & Wang, P. (2010). Research Domain Criteria (RDoC): Toward a new classification framework for research on mental disorders. *American Journal of Psychiatry, 167,* 748–775.

Insel, T., & Quirion, R. (2005). Psychiatry as a clinical neuroscience discipline. *JAMA: The Journal of the American Medical Association, 294,* 2221–2224.

Iwawaki, S., Eysenck, S. B. G., & Eysenck, H. J. (1977). Differences in personality between Japanese and English. *Journal of Social Psychology, 102,* 27–33.

Jacobs, J. (1961). *The death and life of great American cities.* New York, NY: Random House.

Jacobson, N. S., Dobson, K. S., Truax, P. A., Addis, M. E., Koerner, K., Gollan, J. K., Gortner, E., & Prince, S. E. (1996). A component analysis of cognitive-behavioral treatment for depression. *Journal of Consulting and Clinical Psychology, 64,* 295–304.

Jaffee, S. R. (2017). Child maltreatment and risk for psychopathology in childhood and adulthood. *Annual Review of Clinical Psychology, 13,* 525–551.

Jaffee, S. R., Caspi, A., & Moffitt, T. (2004). Physical maltreatment victim to antisocial child: Evidence of an environmentally mediated process.

Journal of Abnormal Psychology, 113, 44–55.

Jaffee, S. R., Moffitt, T. E., Caspi, A., & Taylor, A. (2003). Life with (or without) father: The benefits of living with two biological parents depend on the father's antisocial behavior. *Child Development, 74,* 109–126.

Jaspers, K. (1999). *General psychopathology* (J. Hoenig & M. W. Hamilton, Trans.). Baltimore, MD: Johns Hopkins Press.

Jennings, W. G., & Fox, B. H. (2012). Neighborhood risk and development of antisocial behavior. *American Journal of Community Psychology, 50,* 101–113.

Kagan, J. (1989). *Unstable ideas: Temperament, cognition, and self.* Cambridge MA: Harvard University Press.

(1994). *Galen's prophecy.* New York, NY: Basic.

Kawachi, I., Subramanian, S. V., & Kim, D. (2007). *Social capital and health.* New York, NY: Springer.

Keles, B., McCrae, N., & Grealish, A. (2020). A systematic review: The influence of social media on depression, anxiety and psychological distress in adolescents. *International Journal of Adolescence and Youth, 25*(1), 79–93.

Kendler, K. S., Aggen, S. H., Czjaikowski, N., Roysamb, E., Tambs, K., Torgersen, S., Neale, M. C., & Reichborn-Kjennerud, T. (2008). The structure of genetic and environmental risk factors for DSM-IV personality disorders: A multivariate twin study. *Archives of General Psychiatry, 65,* 1438–1446.

Kerig, P. K., & Stellwagen, K. K. (2010). Roles of callous-unemotional traits, narcissism, and Machiavellianism in childhood aggression. *Journal of Psychopathology and Behavioral Assessment, 32,* 343–352.

Kernberg, O. F. (1976). *Borderline conditions and pathological narcissism.* New York, NY: Jason Aronson.

(1987). *Severe personality disorders.* New York, NY: Basic Books.

Kessler, R. C., Chiu, W. T., Demler, O., Merikangas, K. R., & Walters, E. E. (2005). Prevalence, severity, and comorbidity of 12-month DSM-IV disorders in the National Comorbidity Survey Replication. *Archives of General Psychiatry, 62,* 617–627.

Keyes, K. M., Nicholson, R., & Kinley, J. (2014). Age, period, and cohort effects in psychological distress in the United States and Canada. *American Journal of Epidemiology, 179,* 1216–1227.

Kim-Cohen, J., Caspi, A., Moffitt, T. E., Harrington, H., Milne, B. J., & Poulton, R. (2003). Prior juvenile diagnoses in adults with mental disorder: Developmental follow-back of a prospective-longitudinal cohort. *Archives of General Psychiatry, 60,* 709–717.

Kirmayer, L. J. (1991). The place of culture in psychiatric nosology: Taijin kyofusho and DSM-III-R. *Journal of Nervous and Mental Disease, 179,* 19–28.

Kirmayer, L. J., Brass, G. M., & Tait, C. L. (2000). The mental health of Aboriginal peoples: Transformations of identity and community. *Canadian Journal of Psychiatry, 45,* 607–616.

Kirmayer, L. J., & Young, A. (1998). Culture and somatization: Clinical, epidemiological, and ethnographic perspectives. *Psychosomatic Medicine, 60,* 420–430.

Kirsch, I., Deacon, B. J., Huedo-Medina, T. B., Scoboria, A., & Moore, T. J. (2008). Initial severity and antidepressant benefits: A meta-analysis of data submitted to the Food and Drug Administration. *PLoS Med, 5,* e45.

Kleinman, A., & Good, B. (Eds.). (1985). *Culture and depression: Studies in the anthropology and cross-cultural psychology of affective disorders.* Berkeley: University of California Press.

Klerman, G. L. (1986). Historical perspectives on contemporary schools of psychopathology. In T. Millon & G. L. Klerman (Eds.), *Contemporary psychopathology: Towards the DSM-IV* (pp. 3–28). New York, NY: Guilford.

Klerman, G. L., & Weissman, M. M. (Eds.). (1993). *New applications of the interpersonal therapy of depression.* Washington, DC: American Psychiatric Press.

Knopik, V. S., Neiderhiser, J. M., DeFries, J. C., & Plomin, R. (2016). *Behavioral genetics* (7th ed.). New York, NY: Worth.

Kohut, H. (1970). *The analysis of the self.* New York, NY: International Universities Press.

(1977). *The restoration of the self.* New York, NY: International Universities Press.

Konrath, S. K. (2011). Changes in dispositional empathy in American college students over time: A meta-analysis. *Personality and Social Psychology Review, 15,* 180–198.

Kotov, R., Krueger, R. F., Watson, D., Achenbach, T. M., Althoff, R. R.,

Bagby, R. M., Brown, T. A., Carpenter, W. T., Caspi, A., Clark, L. A., Eaton, N., Forbes, M. K., Forbush, K. T., Goldberg, D., Hasin, D., Hyman, S. E., Ivanova, M. Y., Lynam, D. R., Markon, K., Miller, J. D. et al. (2017). The Hierarchical Taxonomy of Psychopathology (HiTOP): A dimensional alternative to traditional nosologies. *Journal of Abnormal Psychology, 126,* 454–477.

Kraepelin, E. (1919). *Dementia praecox and paraphrenia* (R. M. Barclay, Transl., G. M. Robertson, Ed.). Edinburgh: E. & S. Livingstone.

Krause-Utz, A., Winter, D., Niedtfeld, I., & Schmahl, C. (2014). The latest neuroimaging findings in borderline personality disorder. *Current Psychiatry Reports, 16,* 438–450.

Krueger, R. F., Clark, L. A., Markon, K. E., Derringer, J., Skodol, A. E., & Livesley, W. J. (2011). Deriving an empirical structure of personality pathology for DSM-5. *Journal of Personality Disorders, 25,* 170–191.

Krueger, R. F., Derringer, J., Markon, K., Watson, D., & Skodol, A. E. (2012). Initial construction of a maladaptive personality trait model and inventory for DSM-5. *Psychological Medicine, 42,* 1879–1890.

Lampe, L. (2016). Avoidant personality disorder as a social anxiety phenotype: Risk factors, associations and treatment. *Current Opinion in Psychiatry, 29,* 64–67.

Laporte, L., Paris, J., Bergevin, T., Fraser, R., & Cardin, J. F. (2018). Clinical outcomes of stepped care for the treatment of borderline personality disorder. *Personality and Mental Health, 12,* 252–264.

Lasch, C. (1977). *Haven in a heartless world: The family besieged.* New York, NY: Basic Books.

(1979). *The culture of narcissism.* New York, NY: Warner.

Leighton, D. C., Harding, J. S., & Macklin, D. B. (1963). *The character of danger: Psychiatric symptoms in selected communities.* New York, NY: Basic Books.

Lenzenweger, M. F., Lane, M. C., Loranger, A. W., & Kessler, R. C. (2007). DSM-IV personality disorders in the national comorbidity survey replication. *Biological Psychiatry, 62,* 553–556.

Lesage, A. D., Boyer, R., Grunberg, F., Vanier, C., & Morissette, R. (1994). Suicide and mental disorders: A case control study of young men. *American Journal of Psychiatry, 151,* 1063–1068.

Levy, K. N., Ellison, W. D., & Reynoso, J. S. (2011). A historical review of narcissism and narcissistic personality. In W. K. Campbell & J. Miller (Eds.), *Handbook of narcissism and narcissistic personality disorder* (pp. 3–13). New York, NY: Wiley.

Linehan, M. M. (1993). *Cognitive behavioral therapy of borderline personality disorder.* New York, NY: Guilford.

Littlewood, R. (2002). *Pathologies of the West.* London: Continuum Books.

Livesley, W. J. (2012). Moving beyond specialized therapies for borderline personality disorder: The importance of integrated domain-focused treatment. *Psychodynamic Psychiatry, 40,* 47–74.

Livesley, W. J., Jang, K., Schroeder, M. L., & Jackson, D. N. (1993). Genetic and environmental factors in personality dimensions. *American Journal of Psychiatry, 150,* 1826–1831.

Livesley, W. J., Jang, K. L., & Vernon, P. A. (1998). Phenotypic and genetic structure of traits delineating personality disorder. *Archives of General Psychiatry, 55,* 941–948.

Lofors, J., & Sundquist, K. (2007). Low-linking social capital as a predictor of mental disorders: A cohort study of 4.5 million Swedes. *Social Science & Medicine, 64,* 21–34.

Loranger, A. W., Sartorius, N., Andreoli, A., Berger, P., Buchheim, P., Channabasavanna, S. M., & Regier, D. A. (1994). The International Personality Disorder Examination: The World Health Organization/ Alcohol, Drug Abuse, and Mental Health Administration international pilot study of personality disorders. *Archives of General Psychiatry, 51,* 215–224.

Lövestad, S., Love, J., Vaez, M., Waern, M., Hensing, G., & Krantz, G. (2019). Suicidal ideation and attempts in population-based samples of women: Temporal changes between 1989 and 2015. *BMC Public Health, 19,* 351.

Lukianoff, G., & Haidt, J. (2019). *The coddling of the American mind.* New York, NY: Penguin.

Maccoby, E. E. (2000). Parenting and its effects on children: On reading and misreading behavior genetics. *Annual Review of Psychology, 51,* 11–27.

Maccoby, E. E., & Jacklin, C. N. (1974). *The psychology of sex differences.* Stanford, CA: Stanford University Press.

Malinovsky-Rummell, R., & Hansen, D. J. (1993). Long-term

consequences of physical abuse. *Psychological Bulletin, 114,* 68–79.

Markus, H., & Kitayama, S. (1991). Culture and the self: Implications for cognition, emotion, and motivation. *Psychological Review, 98,* 224–253.

Markus, H. M., & Kitayama, S. (1994). A collective fear of the collective: Implications for selves and theories of selves. *Personality and Social Psychology Bulletin, 20,* 568–579.

Marwick, A. (2000). *The sixties: Cultural revolution in Britain, France, Italy, and the United States, c.1958–c.1974.* New York, NY: Oxford University Press.

McCord, J. (1978). A thirty-year follow-up of treatment effects. *American Psychologist, 33,* 284–289.

McCrae, R. R., & Costa, P. T. (1997). Personality as a human universal. *American Psychologist, 52,* 509–516.

McCrae, R. R., Costa, P. T., & Martin, T. A. (2005). The NEO PI-3: A more readable revised NEO personality inventory. *Journal of Personality Assessment, 84,* 261–270.

McCrae, R. R., & Terracciano, A. (2005). Personality profiles of cultures: Aggregate personality traits. *Journal of Personality & Social Psychology, 89,* 407–425.

McGoldrick, M., Pearce, J. K., & Giordano, J. (1982). *Ethnicity and family therapy.* New York, NY: Guilford.

McKenzie, K. (2008). Urbanization, social capital and mental health. *Global Social Policy, 8,* 359–377.

McKenzie, K., & Harpham, T. (Eds.). (2006). *Social capital and mental health.* London: Jessica Kingsley.

McKenzie, K., Whitley, R., & Weich, S. (2002). Social capital and mental health. *British Journal of Psychiatry, 181,* 280–283.

McMain, S., & Chapman, A. (2019). Results of the FASTER study. Presented to the International Society for the Study of Personality Disorders, Vancouver, Canada, October.

Mednick, S. A., Gabrieli, W. F., & Hutchings, B. (1984). Genetic influences in criminal convictions. *Science, 224,* 891–894.

Mercado, M. C., Holland, K., Leemis, R. W., & Stone, D. M. (2017). Trends in emergency department visits for nonfatal self-inflicted injuries among youth aged 10 to 24 years in the United States, 2001–2015. *JAMA: The Journal of the American Medical Association, 318,* 1931–1933.

Merskey, H. (1997). *The analysis of hysteria* (2nd ed.). London: Royal College of Psychiatrists.

Meyer, A. (1957). *Psychobiology.* Springfield, IL: Charles C. Thomas.

Miller, J. D., & Campbell, W. K. (2010). The case for using research on trait narcissism as a building block for understanding narcissistic personality disorder. *Personality Disorders: Theory, Research, and Treatment, 1,* 180–191.

Miller, J. D., Campbell, W. K., & Pilkonis, P. A. (2007). Narcissistic personality disorder: Relations with distress and functional impairment. *Comprehensive Psychiatry, 48,* 170–177.

Miller, J. D., Dir, A., Gentile, B., Wilson, L., Pryor, L. R., & Campbell, W. K. (2010a). Searching for a vulnerable dark triad: Comparing factor 2 psychopathy, vulnerable narcissism, and borderline personality disorder.

Journal of Personality, 78, 1529–1564.

Miller, J. D., Gaughan, E. T., Pryor, L. R., Kamen, C., & Campbell, W. K. (2009). Is research using the narcissistic personality inventory relevant for understanding narcissistic personality disorder? *Journal of Research in Personality, 43,* 482–488.

Miller, J. D., Hoffman, B. J., Campbell, W. K., & Pilkonis, P. A. (2008). An examination of the factor structure of *Diagnostic and Statistical Manual of Mental Disorders,* Fourth Edition, narcissistic personality disorder criteria: One or two factors? *Comprehensive Psychiatry, 49,* 141–145.

Miller, J. D., & Maples, J. (2011). Trait personality models of narcissistic personality disorder, grandiose narcissism, and vulnerable narcissism. In W. K. Campbell & J. Miller (Eds.), *Handbook of narcissism and narcissistic personality disorder* (pp. 71–88). New York, NY: Wiley.

Miller, J. D., Widiger, T. A., & Campbell, W. K. (2010b). Narcissistic personality disorder and the DSM-V. *Journal of Abnormal Psychology, 119,* 640–649.

Millon, T. (1993). Borderline personality disorder: A psychosocial epidemic. In J. Paris (Ed.), *Borderline personality disorder: Etiology and treatment* (pp. 197–221). Washington, DC: American Psychiatric Press.

Mitchell, K. (2018). *Innate: How the wiring of our brains shapes who we are.* Princeton, NJ: Princeton University Press.

Moffitt, T. E. (2005). The new look of behavioral genetics in developmental psychopathology: Gene–environment interplay in antisocial behaviors. *Psychological Bulletin, 131,* 533–554.

Moffitt, T. E., Caspi, A., Rutter, M., & Silva, P. A. (2001). Sex effects in risk predictors for antisocial behaviour: Are males more vulnerable than females? In T. Moffitt (Ed.), *Sex differences in antisocial behaviour: Conduct disorder, delinquency, and violence in the Dunedin Longitudinal Study* (Cambridge Studies in Criminology, pp. 109–122). Cambridge, UK: Cambridge University Press.

Monroe, S. M., & Simons, A. D. (1991). Diathesis-stress theories in the context of life stress research. *Psychological Bulletin, 110,* 406–425.

Morey, L. C., Hopwood, C. J., Gunderson, J. G., Zanarini, M. C., Skodol, A. E., Shea, M. T., Yen, S., Stout, R. L., Grilo, C. M., Sanislow, C. A., & McGlashan, T. H. (2007). Comparison of diagnostic models for personality disorders. *Psychological Medicine, 37,* 983–994.

Morey, L. C., Skodol, A. E., & Oldham, J. M. (2014). Clinician judgments of clinical utility: A comparison of DSM-IV-TR personality disorders and the alternative model for DSM-5 personality disorders. *Journal of Abnormal Psychology, 123,* 398–405.

Morgan, C., & Kleinman, A. (2010). Social science perspectives: A failure of the sociological imagination. In C. Morgan & D. Bhugra (Eds.), *Principles of social psychiatry* (2nd ed., pp. 51–64). London: Wiley-Blackwell.

Morgan, C., Knowles, G., & Hutchinson, G. (2019). Migration, ethnicity and psychoses: Evidence, models and future direction. *World Psychiatry, 18*, 247–258.

Morgan, C., Webb, R. T., & Carr, M. J. (2017). Incidence, clinical management, and mortality risk following self harm among children and adolescents: Cohort study in primary care. *British Medical Journal, 359*, j4351.

Mulder, R. T. (2004). Depression and personality disorder. *Current Psychiatry Reports, 6*, 51–57.

Murphy, H. B. M. (1982). *Comparative psychiatry*. New York, NY: Springer.

Nandi, D. N., Banerjee, G., Nandi, S., & Nandi, P. (1992). Is hysteria on the wane? *British Journal of Psychiatry, 160*, 87–91.

National Institute for Health and Care Excellence (NICE). (2009). *Borderline personality disorder: Recognition and management*. NICE Guidelines. www.nice.org.uk/guidance/CG78/.

New, A. S., Goodman, M., Triebwasser, J., & Siever, L. J. (2008). Recent advances in the biological study of personality disorders. *Psychiatric Clinics of North America, 31*, 441–461.

Newton-Howes, G., Tyrer, P., & Johnson, T. (2006). Personality disorder and the outcome of depression: Meta-analysis of published studies. *British Journal of Psychiatry, 188*, 13–20.

Nixon, M. K., & Health, N. L. (2008). *Self-injury in youth: The essential guide to assessment and intervention*. New York, NY: Routledge.

Oakley-Browne, M. A., Joyce, P. R., Wells, E., Bushnell, J. A., & Hornblow, A. R. (1989). Christchurch psychiatric epidemiology study: II. Six month and other period prevalences of specific psychiatric disorders. *Australian and New Zealand Journal of Psychiatry, 23*, 327–340.

Ogrodniczuk, J. S., Piper, W. E., Joyce, A. S., Steinberg, P. I., & Duggal, S. (2009). Interpersonal problems associated with narcissism among psychiatric outpatients. *Journal of Psychiatric Research, 43*, 837–842.

Oldham, J. M. (2009). Borderline personality disorder comes of age. *American Journal of Psychiatry, 166*, 509–511.

Olfson, M., Blanco, C., & Wall, M. (2017). Suicidal ideation and attempts in population-based samples of women: Temporal changes between 1989 and 2015. *JAMA Psychiatry, 74*, 1095–1103.

Olfson, M., Marcus, S. C., Druss, B., & Pincus, H. A. (2002). National trends in the use of outpatient psychotherapy. *American Journal of Psychiatry, 159*, 1914–1920.

Oltmanns, J. R., & Widiger, T. A. (2019). Evaluating the assessment of the ICD-11 personality disorder diagnostic system. *Psychological Assessment, 31*, 674–684.

Orben, A., Dienlin, T., & Przybylski, A. (2019). Social media's enduring effect on adolescent life satisfaction. *Proceedings of the National Academy of Sciences, 116*, 10226–10228.

Orlinsky, D. E., Grawe, K., & Parks, B. K. (1994). Process and outcome in psychotherapy: Noch einmal. In A. E. Bergin and S. L. Garfield (Eds.), *Handbook of psychotherapy and behavior change* (pp. 270–379). New York, NY: Wiley.

Otto, M. W., Smits, J., & Reese, H. E. (2006). Combined psychotherapy and pharmacotherapy for mood and anxiety disorders in adults: Review and analysis. *Clinical Psychology: Science and Practice, 12,* 72–86.

Pao, N. P. (1967) The syndrome of deliberate self-cutting. *British Journal of Medical Psychology, 42,* 195–206.

Papageorgiou, K. A., Denovan, A., & Dagnall, N. (2019). The positive effect of narcissism on depressive symptoms through mental toughness: Narcissism may be a dark trait but it does help with seeing the world less grey. *European Psychiatry, 55,* 74–79.

Paris, J. (1996). Cultural factors in the emergence of borderline pathology. *Psychiatry, 59,* 185–192.

(1997). Social factors in the personality disorders. *Transcultural Psychiatry, 34,* 421–452.

(2000). *Myths of childhood.* Philadelphia: Brunner/Mazel.

(2003). *Personality disorders over time: Precursors, course, and outcome.* Washington, DC: American Psychiatric Publishing.

(2004). Sociocultural factors in the treatment of personality disorders. In J. J. Magnavita (Ed.), *Handbook of personality disorders: Theory and practice* (pp. 135–147). Hoboken, NJ: Wiley.

(2008). Clinical trials in personality disorders. *Psychiatric Clinics of North America, 31,* 517–526.

(2010a). Effectiveness of differing psychotherapy approaches in the treatment of borderline personality disorder. *Current Psychiatry Reports, 12,* 56–60.

(2010b). Estimating the prevalence of personality disorders. *Journal of Personality Disorders, 24,* 405–411.

(2013). *Psychotherapy in an age of narcissism.* London: Palgrave MacMillan.

(2014). Modernity and narcissistic personality disorder. *Personality Disorders: Theory, Research, and Treatment, 5,* 220–226.

(2015). *A concise guide to personality disorders.* Washington, DC: American Psychological Association.

(2020). *The treatment of borderline personality disorder: An evidence-based approach.* New York, NY: Guilford.

Paris, J., & Kirmayer, L. (2016). The NIMH research domain criteria: A bridge too far. *Journal of Nervous and Mental Diseases, 204,* 26–32.

Paris, J., & Lis, E. (2013). Can sociocultural and historical mechanisms influence the development of borderline personality disorder? *Transcultural Psychiatry, 50,* 140–151.

Paris, J., & Zweig-Frank, H. (2001). A 27 year follow-up of patients with borderline personality disorder. *Comprehensive Psychiatry, 42,* 482–487.

Patel, V. (2001). Cultural factors and international epidemiology: Depression and public health. *British Medical Bulletin, 57,* 33–45.

Parker, G. (1983). *Parental overprotection: A risk factor in psychosocial development.* New York, NY: Grune & Stratton.

Parker, G., & Brotchie, H. (2010). Gender differences in depression. *International Review of Psychiatry, 22,* 429–436.

Paykel, E. S., Abbott, R., Jenkins, R., Brugha, T. S., & Meltzer, H. (2000) Urban-rural mental health differences in Great Britain: Findings from the National Morbidity Survey. *Psychological Medicine, 30,* 269–280.

Peen, J., Schoevers, R. A., Beekman, A. T., & Dekker, J. (2010). The current status of urban–rural differences in psychiatric disorders. *Acta Psychiatrica Scandinavica, 121,* 84–93.

Pies, R. (2011). How to eliminate narcissism overnight: DSM-V and the death of narcissistic personality disorder. *Innovations in Clinical Neuroscience, 8,* 23–27.

Pike, K. M., & Dunne, P. E. (2015). The rise of eating disorders in Asia: A review. *Journal of Eating Disorders, 3,* 33–40.

Pincus, A. L., Ansell, E. B., Pimentel, C., Cain, N. M., Wright, A. G., & Levy, K. L. (2009). Initial construction and validation of the Pathological Narcissism Inventory. *Psychological Assessment, 21,* 365–379.

Pincus, A. L., & Lukowitsky, M. R. (2010). Pathological narcissism and narcissistic personality disorder. *Annual Review of Clinical Psychology, 6,* 421–446.

Pinker, S. (2011). *The better angels of our nature: Why violence has declined.* New York, NY: Viking.
    (2018). *Enlightenment now.* New York, NY: Penguin.

Pinto, C., Dhavale, D., Hemangee, S., Nair, S., Patil, B., & Dewan, C. (2000). Borderline personality disorder exists in India. *The Journal of Nervous and Mental Disease, 188,* 386–388.

Plomin, R., & Bergeman, C. (1991). Genetic influence on environmental measures. *Behavioral and Brain Sciences, 14,* 373–427.

Pollock, V. E., Briere, J., Schneider, L., Knop, J., Mednick, S. A., & Goodwin, D. W. (1990). Childhood antecedents of antisocial behavior: Parental alcoholism and physical abusiveness. *American Journal of Psychiatry, 147,* 1290–1293.

Prince, R., & Tseng-Laroche, F. (1990). Culture-bound syndromes and international disease classification. *Culture, Medicine, and Psychiatry, 11,* 1–49.

Putnam, R. D. (2000). *Bowling alone: The collapse and revival of American community.* New York, NY: Simon & Schuster.

Raine, A. (2013). *The anatomy of violence: The biological roots of crime.* New York, NY: Random House.

Ranger, M., Tyrer, P., Miloseska, K., Fourie, H., Khaleel, I., North, B., & Barrett, B. (2009). Cost-effectiveness of nidotherapy for comorbid personality disorder and severe mental illness: Randomized controlled trial. *Epidemiologia e Psichiatria Sociale, 18,* 128–136.

Raskin, R., & Terry, H. (1988). A principal-components analysis of the Narcissistic Personality Inventory and further evidence of its construct validity. *Journal of Personality and Social Psychology, 54*(5), 890–902.

Reich, W. (1933/1990). *Character analysis* (V. R. Carfagno, Trans.). New York, NY: Farrar, Strauss & Giroux.

Reichborn-Kjennerud, T., Ystrom, E., Neale, M. C., Aggen, S. H., Mazzeo,

S. E., Knudsen, G. P., Tambs, K., Czajkowski, N. O., & Kendler, K. S. (2013). Structure of genetic and environmental risk factors for symptoms of DSM-IV borderline personality disorder. *JAMA Psychiatry, 70,* 1206–1214.

Rey, J. M., Singh, M., Morris-Yates, A., & Andrews, G. (1997). Referred adolescents as young adults: The relationship between psychosocial functioning and personality disorder. *Australian and New Zealand Journal of Psychiatry, 31,* 219–226.

Richerson, P. J., & Boyd, R. (2006). *Not by genes alone: How culture transformed human evolution.* Chicago: University of Chicago Press.

Rieff, P. (1966). *The triumph of the therapeutic: Uses of faith after Freud.* New York, NY: Harper & Row.

Riley, G. (1991). *Divorce: An American tradition.* New York, NY: Oxford University Press.

Rioux, C., Seguin, J., & Paris, J. (2018). Differential susceptibility to the environment and borderline personality disorder. *Harvard Review of Psychiatry, 2,* 374–380.

Robins, L. N. (1966). *Deviant children grown up.* Baltimore, MD: Williams and Wilkins.

Robins, L. N., & Regier, D. A. (1991). *Psychiatric disorders in America.* New York, NY: Free Press.

Rodgers, J. L., Rowe, D. C., & Buster, M. (1998). Social contagion, adolescent sexual behavior, and pregnancy: A nonlinear dynamic EMOSA model. *Developmental Psychology, 34,* 1096–1113.

Rogers, C. (1951). *Client-centered therapy: Its current practice,* *implications and theory.* London: Constable.

Ronningstam, E. (2009). Narcissistic personality disorder: A current review. *Current Psychiatry Reports, 12,* 68–75.

(2011). Narcissistic personality disorder: A clinical perspective. *Journal of Psychiatric Practice, 17,* 89–99.

Rosenthal, S. A., & Hooley, J. M. (2010). Narcissism assessment in social–personality research: Does the association between narcissism and psychological health result from a confound with self-esteem? *Journal of Research in Personality, 44,* 453–465.

Rosenthal, S. A., Montoya, R. M., Ridings, L. E., Rieck, S. M., & Hooley, J. M. (2011). Further evidence of the Narcissistic Personality Inventory's validity problems: A meta-analytic investigation – Response to Miller, Maples, and Campbell. *Journal of Personality, 45,* 408–416.

Rossier, J., Rigozzi, C., & Personality Across Culture Research Group. (2008). Personality disorders and the five-factor model among French speakers in Africa and Europe. *Canadian Journal of Psychiatry, 53,* 534–544.

Rothbart, M. (2011). *Becoming who we are: Temperament and personality in development.* New York, NY: Guilford.

Rutter, M. (1971). Parent-child separation: Psychological effects on the children. *Journal of Child Psychology and Psychiatry, 12,* 233–260.

(1987). Temperament, personality, and personality development. *British Journal of Psychiatry, 150,* 443–448.

(1989). Pathways from childhood to adult life. *Journal of Child Psychology & Psychiatry, 30*, 23–51.

(2006). *Genes and behavior: Nature-nurture interplay explained.* London: Blackwell.

(2012). Resilience as a dynamic concept. *Development and Psychopathology, 24*, 335–344.

Rutter, M., & Maughan, B. (1997). Psychosocial adversities in psychopathology. *Journal of Personality Disorders, 11*, 19–33.

Rutter, M., & Rutter, M. (1993). *Developing minds: Challenge and continuity across the life span.* London: Penguin.

Rutter, M., & Smith, D. J. (1995). *Psychosocial problems in young people.* Cambridge, UK: Cambridge University Press.

Sameroff, A. J. (1995). General systems theories and developmental psychopathology. In D. Cicchetti and D. J. Cohen (Eds.), *Developmental psychopathology: Theory and methods* (pp. 659–699). New York, NY: John Wiley.

Satel, S., & Sommers, C. H. (2005). *One nation under therapy: How the helping culture is eroding self-reliance.* New York, NY: St. Martin's Press.

Sato, T., & Takeichi, D. (1993). Lifetime prevalence of specific psychiatric disorders in a general medicine clinic. *General Hospital Psychiatry, 15*, 224–233.

Scarr, S., & McCartney, K. (1983). How people make their own environments: A theory of genotype-environment effects. *Child Development, 54*, 424–435.

Schacter, D. L. (1996). *Searching for memory. The brain, the mind, and the past.* New York, NY: Basic Books.

Scheff, T. (1989). *Being mentally ill: A sociological theory* (3rd ed.). Chicago: Aldine Press.

Schneider, K. (1950). *Psychopathic personalities* (9th ed.). London: Cassell.

Schofield, T. J., Conger, R. D., Conger, K. J., Martin, M. J., Brody, G., Simons, R., & Cutrona, S. (2012). The protective effect of family support among Mexican American and African American families. *American Journal of Community Psychology, 50*, 101–113.

Senol, S., Dereboy, C., & Yüksel, N. (1997) Borderline disorder in Turkey: A 2- to 4-year follow-up. *Social Psychiatry and Psychiatric Epidemiology, 32*, 109–112.

Sharpley, M., Hutchinson, G., McKenzie, K., & Murray, R. M. (2001). Understanding the excess of psychosis among the African-Caribbean population in England: Review of current hypotheses. *British Journal of Psychiatry, 40*, s60–68.

Shorter, E. (1992). *From paralysis to fatigue.* New York, NY: Wiley.

(1997). *A history of psychiatry.* New York, NY: Wiley.

Siever, L. J., & Davis, K. L. (1991). A psychobiological perspective on the personality disorders. *American Journal of Psychiatry, 148*, 1647–1658.

Skodol, A. E., Gunderson, J. G., Shea, M. T., McGlashan, T. H., Morey, L. C., & Sanislow, C. A. (2005). The Collaborative Longitudinal Personality Disorders Study (CLPS): Overview and implications. *Journal of Personality Disorders, 19*, 487–504.

Snyder, J. (2015). Coercive family processes in the development of externalizing behavior: Incorporating neurobiology into intervention research. In T. P. Beauchaine & S. P. Hinshaw (Eds.), *The Oxford handbook of externalizing spectrum disorders* (pp. 286–315). New York, NY: Oxford University Press.

Song, L. (2011). Social capital and psychological distress. *Journal of Health and Social Behavior, 52,* 478–492.

Srole, L., & Fischer, A. K. (1980). The Midtown Manhattan Longitudinal Study vs. "The Mental Paradise Lost Doctrine." *Archives of General Psychiatry, 37,* 209–218.

Stein, M. B., Jang, K., & Livesley, W. J. (2002). Heritability of social anxiety-related concerns and personality characteristics: A twin study. *Journal of Nervous and Mental Disease, 190,* 219–224.

Stepp, S. D., Lazarus, S. A., & Byrd, A. L. (2016). A systematic review of risk factors prospectively associated with borderline personality disorder: Taking stock and moving forward. *Personality Disorders: Theory, Research, and Treatment, 7,* 316–323.

Stern, A. (1938). Psychoanalytic investigation of and therapy in the borderline group of neuroses. *Psychoanalytic Quarterly, 7,* 467–489.

Stinson, F. S., Dawson, D. A., Goldstein, R. B., Chou, S. P., Huang, B., & Smith, S. M. (2008). Prevalence, correlates, disability, and comorbidity of personality disorder diagnoses in a DSM-IV narcissistic personality disordered non-patient sample: Results from the wave 2 national epidemiologic survey on alcohol and related conditions. *Journal of Clinical Psychiatry, 69,* 1033–1045.

Stoffers, J., Völlm, B. A., Rücker, G., Timmer, A., Huband, N., & Lieb, K. (2010). Pharmacological interventions for borderline personality disorder. *Cochrane Database of Systematic Reviews, (6),* CD005653.

Stone, M. H. (1993). *Abnormalities of personality.* New York, NY: Norton.

(1997). *Healing the mind: A history of psychiatry from antiquity to the present.* New York, NY: Norton.

Sullivan, F. C. (2010). The Psychiatric GWAS Consortium: Big science comes to psychiatry. *Neuron, 68,* 182–186.

Sutker, P. B., Bugg, F., & West, J. A. (1993). Antisocial personality disorder. In P. B. Sutker & H. E. Adams (Eds.), *Comprehensive textbook of psychopathology* (pp. 337–369). New York, NY: Plenum.

Tackett, J. L., & Mackrell, S. (2011). Narcissism and Machiavellianism in youth: Implications for the development of adaptive and maladaptive behavior. In C. T. Barry, P. K. Kerig, & K. K. Stellwagen (Eds.), *Narcissism and Machiavellianism in youth* (pp. 11–23). Washington, DC: American Psychological Association.

Taiminen, T. J., Kallio-Soukainen, K., Nokso-Koivisto, H., Kaljonen, A., & Helenius, H. (1998). Contagion of deliberate self-harm among adolescent inpatients. *Journal of the American Academy of Child & Adolescent Psychiatry, 37,* 211–217.

Taylor, C. (1992). *The malaise of modernity.* Toronto: Anisna.

Tew, J. (2012). Recovery capital: What enables a sustainable recovery from mental health difficulties? *European Journal of Social Work, 16*(3), 360–374.

Tew, J., Ramon, S., Slade, M., Bird, V., & Melton, J. (2011). Social factors and recovery from mental health difficulties: A review of the evidence. *British Journal of Social Work, 15*, 1–18.

Thomaes, S., Stegge, H., Bushman, B. J., Olthof, T., & Denissen, J. (2008). Development and validation of the Childhood Narcissism Scale. *Journal of Personality Assessment, 90*(4), 382–391.

Tirupati, S., Conrad, A., Frost, B., & Johnston, S. (2010). Urban–rural differences in psychiatric rehabilitation outcomes. *Australian Journal of Rural Health, 18*, 66–71.

Tocqueville, A. de (1835/2000). *Democracy in America* (H. Mansfield & D. Winthrop, Trans. and Eds.). Chicago: University of Chicago Press.

Tonnies, F. (1974). *On social ideas and ideologies* (E. G. Jacoby, Trans., Ed., and annotated by). New York, NY: Harper & Row.

Topor, A., Borg, M., Girolamo, S., & Davidson, L. (2011). Not just an individual journey: Social aspects of recovery. *International Journal of Social Psychiatry, 57*, 90–99.

Torgersen, S. (2009). The nature (and nurture) of personality disorders. *Scandinavian Journal of Psychology, 50*, 624–632.

Torgersen, S., Kringlen, E., & Cramer, V. (2001). The prevalence of personality disorders in a community sample. *Archives of General Psychiatry, 58*, 590–596.

Torgersen, S., Lygren, S., Oien, P. A., Skre, I., Onstad, S., Edvardsen, J., Tambs, K., & Kringlen, E. (2000). A twin study of personality disorders. *Comprehensive Psychiatry, 41*, 416–425.

Torgersen, S., Myers, J., Reichborn-Kjennerud, T., Røysamb, E., Kubarych, T. S., & Kendler, K. S. (2012). The heritability of Cluster B personality disorders assessed both by personal interview and questionnaire. *Journal of Personality Disorders, 26*, 848–866.

Torrey, E. F. (1992). *Freudian fraud.* New York, NY: Harper Perennial.

Trull, T. J. (2014). Ruminations on narcissistic personality disorder. *Personality Disorders: Theory, Research, and Treatment, 5*, 230–231.

Trull, T. J., Jahng, S., Tomko, R. L., Wood, P. K., & Sher, K. J. (2010). Revised NESARC personality disorder diagnoses: Gender, prevalence, and comorbidity with substance dependence disorders. *Journal of Personality Disorders, 24*, 412–426.

Trzesniewski, K. H., Donnellan, M. B., & Robins, R. W. (2008a). Do today's young people really think they are so extraordinary? An examination of secular changes in narcissism and self-enhancement. *Psychological Science, 19*, 181–188.

(2008b). Is "Generation Me" really more narcissistic than previous generations? *Journal of Personality, 76*, 903–917.

Tseng, W. T. (Ed.). (2001). *Handbook of cultural psychiatry.* New York, NY: Academic Press.

Twenge, J. M. (2011). Culture and narcissism. In W. K. Campbell & J. Miller (Eds.), *Handbook of narcissism and narcissistic personality disorder* (pp. 202–209). New York, NY: Wiley.

(2013). Does online social media lead to social connection or social disconnection? *Journal of College and Character, 14,* 11–20.

Twenge, J. M., & Campbell, W. K. (2009). *The narcissism epidemic: Living in the age of entitlement.* New York, NY: Simon & Schuster.

(2018). Associations between screen time and lower psychological well-being among children and adolescents: Evidence from a population-based study. *Preventative Medicine Reports, 12,* 271–283.

Twenge, J. M., Cooper, A. B., Joiner, T. E., Duffy, M. E., & Binau, S. G. (2019). Age, period, and cohort trends in mood disorder indicators and suicide-related outcomes in a nationally representative dataset, 2005–2017. *Journal of Abnormal Psychology, 128,* 185–199.

Twenge, J. M., Joiner, T. E., Rogers, M. L., & Martin, G. N. (2017). Increases in depressive symptoms, suicide-related outcomes, and suicide rates among U.S. adolescents after 2010 and links to increased new media screen time. *Clinical Psychological Science, 6,* 3–17.

Tyrer, P. (2008). Nidotherapy: A new approach to the treatment of personality disorder. *Acta Psychiatrica Scandinavica, 105,* 469–471.

(2009). Why borderline personality disorder is neither borderline nor a personality disorder. *Personality and Mental Health, 3,* 86–95.

Tyrer, P., Crawford, M., Mulder, R., Blashfield, R., Farnam, A., Fossati, A., Kim, Y.-R., Koldobsky, N., Lecic-Tosevski, D., Ndetei, D., Swales, M., Clark, L. A., & Reed, G. M. (2011a). The rationale for the reclassification of personality disorder in the 11th revision of the *International Classification of Diseases* (ICD-11). *Personality and Mental Health, 5,* 246–259.

Tyrer, P., Miloseska, K., Whittington, C., Ranger, M., Khaleel, I., & Crawford, M. (2011b). Nidotherapy in the treatment of substance misuse, psychosis and personality disorder: Secondary analysis of a controlled trial. *The Psychiatrist, 35,* 9–14.

Tyrer, P., Tarabi, S. A., Bassett, P., Liedtka, N., Hall, R., Nagar, J., Imrie, A., & Tyrer, H. (2017). Nidotherapy compared with enhanced care programme approach training for adults with aggressive challenging behaviour and intellectual disability (NIDABID): Cluster randomised controlled trial. *Journal of Intellectual Disability Research, 61,* 521–531.

Tyrer, P., & Tyrer, H. (2018). *Nidotherapy: Harmonising the environment with the patient.* London: Royal College of Psychiatrists.

Vaddadi, K. (2010). Rehabilitation psychiatry: Moving forward. *International Review of Psychiatry, 22,* 95–98.

Vaillant, G. E. (1977). *Adaptation to life.* Cambridge, MA: Little, Brown.

Vaillant, G. E., & Vaillant, C. O. (1981). Natural history of male psychological health X: Work as a predictor of positive mental health.

American Journal of Psychiatry, 138, 1433–1438.

VanZomeren-Dohm, K., Xu, X., Thibodeau, E., & Cicchetti, D. (2015). Child maltreatment and vulnerability to externalizing spectrum disorders. In T. P. Beauhaine & S. P. Hinshaw (Eds.), *The Oxford handbook of externalizing spectrum disorders* (pp. 267–298). New York, NY: Oxford University Press.

Verheul, R., Bartak, A., & Widiger, T. (2007). Prevalence and construct validity of Personality Disorder Not Otherwise Specified (PDNOS). *Journal of Personality Disorders, 21,* 359–370.

Vernon, P. A., Villani, V. C., Vickers, L. C., & Harris, J. A. (2008). A behavioral genetic investigation of the Dark Triad and the Big 5. *Personality and Individual Differences, 44,* 445–452.

Wallerstein, J. (1989). *Second chances: Men, women, and children a decade after divorce.* New York, NY: Ticknor and Fields.

Walsh, Z., Shea, T., Yen, S., Ansell, E. B., & Gunderson, J. G. (2012). Socioeconomic-status and mental health in a personality disorder sample: The importance of neighborhood factors. *Journal of Personality Disorders, 26,* 61–64.

Wampold, B. E. (2001). *The great psychotherapy debate: Models, methods, and findings.* Mahwah, NJ: Erlbaum.

Weinbrecht, A., Schulze, L., Boettcher, J., & Renneberg, B. (2016). Avoidant personality disorder: A current review. *Current Psychiatry Reports, 18,* 29–40.

Weissman, M. M., & Olfson, M. (1995). Depression in women: Implications for health care research. *Science, 269,* 799–801.

Weissman, R. S. (2019). The role of sociocultural factors in the etiology of eating disorders. *Psychiatric Clinics of North America, 42,* 121–140.

Weisz, J. R., Sigman, M., Weiss, B., & Mosk, J. (1993). Parent reports of behavioral and emotional problems among children in Kenya, Thailand, and the United States. *Child Development, 64,* 98–109.

Welander-Vatn, A., Torvik, F., Czajkowski, N., Kendler, K. S., Reichborn-Kjennerud, T., Knudsen, G., & Ystrom, E. (2019). Relationships among avoidant personality disorder, social anxiety disorder, and normative personality traits: A twin study. *Journal of Personality Disorders, 33,* 289–309.

Werner, E. E., & Smith, R. S. (1992). *Overcoming the odds: High risk children from birth to adulthood.* Ithaca, NY: Cornell University Press.

Werner, K. B., Few, L. R., & Bucholz, K. K. (2015). Epidemiology, comorbidity, and behavioral genetics of antisocial personality disorder and psychopathy. *Psychiatric Annals, 45,* 195–199.

Wertz, J., Agnew-Blais, J., Caspi, A., Fisher, H. L., & Moffitt, T. E. (2018). From childhood conduct problems to poor functioning at age 18 years: Examining explanations in a longitudinal cohort study. *Journal of the American Academy of Child & Adolescent Psychiatry, 57,* 54–60.

West, D. J., & Farrington, D. P. (1973). *Who becomes delinquent?* London: Heinemann.

Westen, D. (1985). *Self and society.* Cambridge, UK: Cambridge University Press.

Westphal, M., & Bonnano, G. A. (2007). Posttraumatic growth and resilience to trauma: Different sides of the same coin or different coins? *Applied Psychology, 56,* 417–427.

Wexler, B. E. (2006). *Brain and culture: Neurobiology, ideology, and social change.* Cambridge, MA: MIT Press.

Witt, S. H., Streit, F., Jungkunz, M., Frank, J., Awasthi, S., Reinbold, C. S., Treutlein, J., Degenhardt, F., Forstner, A. J., Heilmann-Heimbach, S., Dietl, L., Schwarze, C. E., Schendel, D., Strohmaier, J., Abdellaoui, A., Adolfsson, R., Air, T. M., Akil, H., Alda, M., Alliey-Rodriguez, N. et al. (2017). Genome-wide association study of borderline personality disorder reveals genetic overlap with bipolar disorder, major depression and schizophrenia. *Translational Psychiatry, 7,* e1155.

Wolfe, T. (1976, August 23). The "Me" decade and the third great awakening. *New York Magazine.*

Woolcock, M. (1998). Social capital and economic development: Towards a theoretical synthesis and policy framework. *Theory and Society, 27,* 151–208.

World Health Organization. (2019). *International classification of diseases* (11th ed.). Geneva: World Health Organization.

Zakinofsky, I., & Roberts, R. (1987). The ecology of suicide in the provinces of Canada. In B. Cooper (Ed.), *The epidemiology of psychiatric disorders* (pp. 27–42). Baltimore, MD: Johns Hopkins University Press.

Zanarini, M. C. (Ed.). (2005). *Textbook of borderline personality disorder.* Philadelphia: Taylor & Francis.

Zanarini, M. C., Frankenburg, F. R., Reich, D. B., & Fitzmaurice, G. (2012). Attainment and stability of sustained symptomatic remission and recovery among patients with borderline personality disorder and Axis II comparison subjects: A 16-year prospective follow-up study. *American Journal of Psychiatry, 169,* 476–483.

Zanor, C. (2010, November 30). A fate that narcissists will hate: Being ignored. *The New York Times.* www.nytimes.com/2010/11/30/ health/views/30mind.html.

Zhong, J., & Leung, F. (2007). Should borderline personality disorder be included in the fourth edition of the Chinese classification of mental disorders? *Chinese Medical Journal, 120,* 77–82.

Zimmerman, M., Balling, C., Dalrymple, K., & Chelminski, I. (2019). Screening for borderline personality disorder in psychiatric outpatients with major depressive disorder and bipolar disorder. *Journal of Clinical Psychiatry, 80*(1), 18m12257.

Zimmerman, M., Rothschild, L., & Chelminski, I. (2005). The prevalence of DSM-IV personality disorders in psychiatric outpatients. *American Journal of Psychiatry, 162,* 1911–1918.

Zoccolillo, M., Pickles, A., Quinton, D., & Rutter, M. (1992). The outcome of childhood conduct disorder: Implications for defining adult personality disorder and conduct disorder. *Psychological Medicine, 22,* 971–986.

Index